Weight Control:
The Medical Reality

Weight Control:
The Medical Reality

R. Bhanot M.D., Ph.D.

iUniverse, Inc.
New York Lincoln Shanghai

Weight Control: The Medical Reality

All Rights Reserved © 2003 by Dr Raj Bhanot

No part of this book may be reproduced or transmitted in any form or by any means, graphic, electronic, or mechanical, including photocopying, recording, taping, or by any information storage retrieval system, without the written permission of the publisher.

iUniverse, Inc.

For information address:
iUniverse, Inc.
2021 Pine Lake Road, Suite 100
Lincoln, NE 68512
www.iuniverse.com

ISBN: 0-595-28103-6

Printed in the United States of America

This book is dedicated to my wife and children.

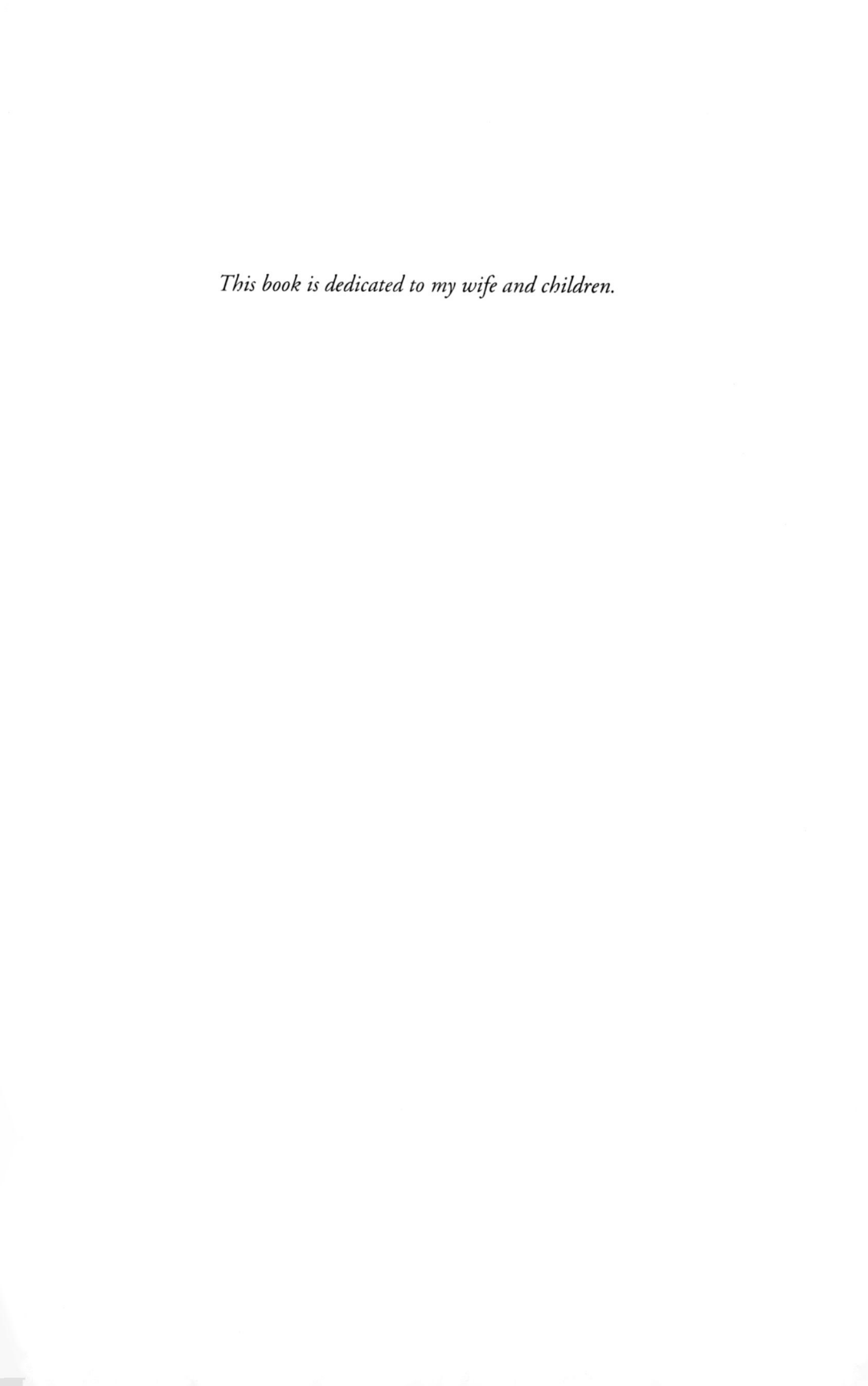

Contents

Introduction xiii
About the Author xvii
A Note on the Use of This Book. xix

CHAPTER 1   Assessment of Body Weight. 1
- *Body mass index. 1*
- *Waist size 3*
- *Overweight children. 4*
- *Body configuration. 4*
- *Recognizing denial. 5*
- *Advantages of being overweight. 6*
- *Case history 7*
- *Comment 8*

CHAPTER 2   Problems with Some Weight Control Strategies 9
- *Commercial programs. 9*
- *Vegetarian diets. 11*
- *Weight cycling 15*
- *Anorexia and bulimia 15*
- *Case history 16*
- *Comment 17*

CHAPTER 3   Getting Started 18
- *Ruling out physical problems. 18*
- *The physician's role 21*
- *Case history 21*

- *Comment* 22

Chapter 4   Energy Balance 23
- *The calorie* 23
- *Using the energy equation* 23
- *Daily energy requirements* 24
- *Calories in fast food* 25
- *Food records* 26
- *Nutrition and weight* 26
- *Case history* 27
- *Comment* 28

Chapter 5   Physical Activity 30
- *Energy expenditure* 30
- *Active lifestyle* 30
- *Exercise guidelines* 32
- *Television and computers* 33
- *Deconditioning* 35
- *Early benefits* 36
- *Case history* 37
- *Comment* 39

Chapter 6   Practical Strategies for Weight Control 40
- *Food labels* 40
- *Lack of results* 42
- *The hunger instinct* 42
- *Dietary fat* 43
- *Very fatty foods* 44
- *Saturated fats* 45
- *Salt consumption* 47
- *Dairy products* 47
- *Calcium and vitamin D* 49
- *Passive strategies* 50
- *Restaurant dinners* 52

- *Sugar consumption* 52
- *Healthier fats* 54
- *Desserts* 55

CHAPTER 7 Weight Control and Diabetes 56
- *The metabolic syndrome* 56
- *Diabetes* 57
- *Case history* 61
- *Comment* 62

CHAPTER 8 Alcohol and Tobacco 63
- *Alcohol* 63
- *Brain chemistry* 63
- *The burden to society* 64
- *Alcohol and energy* 66
- *Tobacco* 67
- *Disorders related to tobacco* 67
- *Nicotine and body weight* 68
- *Case history* 69
- *Comment* 70

CHAPTER 9 Medical Implications of Lifestyle Changes 71
- *Initial screening* 71
- *Heart disease* 72
- *Monitoring the pulse* 73
- *Lipids* 75
- *The Mediterranean diet* 76
- *Osteoarthritis* 77
- *Outdoor physical activity* 80
- *Longevity* 81
- *Personal priorities* 82

CHAPTER 10 Glossary of Medical Terms 84
CHAPTER 11 List of References 92

Acknowledgements

I am indebted to Ian Cameron M.D., CCFP, professor, Department of Family Medicine, Dalhousie University, Halifax, Nova Scotia; and to Michael Ackermann M.D., staff physician, St. Mary's Memorial Hospital, Sherbrooke, Nova Scotia, for reviewing the manuscript and making helpful comments. I would also like to thank Ms. Tina Witherall Pdt, CDE, staff dietitian, St. Mary's Memorial Hospital, Sherbrooke, and Guysborough Memorial Hospital, Guysborough, Nova Scotia, for her expert advice regarding nutrition-related issues. I am also grateful to those individuals who have provided their thoughts about lifestyle issues, which appear with permission. This project would not have been possible without computer support provided by my son.

Introduction

Weight Control: The Medical Reality was written in order to provide basic medical information to the general reader pertaining to the maintenance of body weight and associated lifestyle issues. It contains information about weight loss as well. However, the book is of equal use to slimmer individuals, since it highlights and discusses issues that are relevant to everyday living. If we believe that an individual can gain one pound a year without any consequences, we would observe a weight gain of forty pounds as one ages from young adulthood to late middle age. This person will need to be aware of many of the principles discussed in this book in order to prevent this. It is clearly better to avoid gaining excessive weight in the first place than trying to lose it later.

Some individuals have complained that they obtained a lot of information from the medical profession regarding prevention *after* developing weight problems, high blood pressure, heart disease or diabetes but not prior to their medical diagnosis, when they actually needed it. This book will address this concern as well.

Although the discussion has medical overtones, it is based on personal experience also. The text is derived not only from medical information and clinical practice but also from my own experiences with lifestyle issues. Likewise, I have drawn from my role as a parent.

In some cases, I have examined accepted medical recommendations from unusual aspects. The new points are medically relevant, but not discussed as widely. The book also provides facts and figures pertaining to information provided by health-caregivers. I have not provided a new dietary regimen or exercise program designed to meet the consumer's needs. I do not think anything of this nature exists. Physicians take a much broader approach when dealing with nutrition and lifestyle issues.

I have avoided writing about the causes of obesity. I believe that there is still considerable disagreement among researchers, who variously consider it a learned behavior, an abnormality in the brain's appetite center, a derangement in circulating appetite hormones, a genetic disorder, a disorder triggered by excessive consumption of carbohydrates, or a problem with the number of fat cells established in developmental stages. Some feel it is related to excessive consumption of food energy, while others believe it is due to a reduction in physical activity.

It is important to appreciate that basic human physiology has not changed in the new millennium compared to thirty or forty years ago, when obesity was less prevalent. Clearly, external factors are involved. Similarly, obesity has remarkable correlations with socioeconomic factors: it is found in wealthier people in developing nations but in lower-income individuals of affluent countries. In this manner, obesity has economic, demographic, social, psychological, and medical aspects. This book provides insight into the last component only.

I have avoided quoting too many statistics, which are commonly cited in the media, since this is not the type of information one expects from discussion with a physician. Instead, we look for ideas and strategies that one can apply on a daily basis. I try to avoid miring the reader in the controversies of nutritional science for the same reasons. I do not deal with the subject of treatment with medications, because this conflicts with the objectives of the book.

I have included some medical vocabulary that is used commonly. Not only is this important to gain a deeper understanding of the issues at hand, but it will also assist discussions with members of the health-care team. I just hope that I have explained the terms adequately. If you find that some terms need clarification, refer to the glossary at the end of the book.

There is also a list of references at the end of the book that identifies some of the research that forms the basis of medical opinion. I have selected fairly current articles published in peer-reviewed journals. I have shown preference for review articles published by experts in their field of research. This is an excellent starting point if you wish to study these matters further. Do not be discouraged if you find that medical findings change over time. Physicians are interested in the medical evidence underlying health recommendations, and this information is being reviewed constantly. Some inconsistency in medical opinion should not persuade clients to abandon their goals or turn to completely unfounded claims.

The reader is encouraged to explore the problem of surrogate markers in medical reasoning. I have attempted to select evidence that is meaningful in terms of increased life expectancy and improved health benefits. For example, medical research has associated the consumption of fish with improvements in life expectancy. This property has been attributed to the presence of particular fats in fish. Eggs that contain these fats are now widely available as well. However, is there evidence that the consumption of these modified eggs results in fewer heart attacks or improved survival? This is a separate issue that would have to be addressed with further research. This problem is commonly encountered when new medications are tested. A new agent may be very effective in lowering blood pressure, but we may discover that it results in more deaths due to factors that were unpredictable. There would be a lack of benefit to patients and physicians would reject the treatment. In these examples, the presence of healthy fats, and the measurement of reduced blood pressures, are encouraging properties. Researchers will need to assess whether or not important clinical problems such as heart attacks, kidney failure, and life expectancy are improved.

The text is organized using chapter and sectional headings to help highlight important points. You can refer to specific sections without losing some of the flow. I have tried to limit the information to general medical principles. Obviously, I cannot give specific advice for individual health concerns without the proper background information. This can be achieved only through the involvement of an appropriate health-care team.

Always remember that the doctor or dietitian is not going to control their client's lifestyle or body weight; the individual bears the ultimate responsibility for these decisions. In order to make these decisions, the client is going to require information that is both reliable and practical, advice that will be useful today and several years in the future. This is the main role these health professionals serve.

I hope that you find this book useful and informative.

R. Bhanot M.D., Ph.D.
June 2003

About the Author

Dr. Bhanot is chief of staff at St. Mary's Memorial Hospital, Sherbrooke, Nova Scotia. He obtained a Ph.D. in medical physiology in 1983 and his medical degree in 1988 in Halifax, Nova Scotia. He has published several research articles dealing with brain research and hormonal control of maturation and reproduction. Recent publications have focused on clinical medicine. This book is for a general readership and is based on his medical training as well as his clinical and personal experiences.

Dr. Bhanot has an active practice dealing with family medicine and hospitalized patients. He is married and has two children, aged sixteen and twelve.

A Note on the Use of This Book

This book was written for information, reference, and discussion purposes only. It can be used as an aid in discussions between patients and their caregivers. It is not meant to replace personal medical advice given by physicians. The information contained herein does not qualify anyone to provide medical advice to others. It represents the author's personal and professional opinions. The author, his executors, and his affiliates cannot be held responsible for any injuries or losses related to the use of this book, however caused.

1

Assessment of Body Weight

BODY MASS INDEX

What do you know about your current weight? It is often inappropriate to use fashion models in television advertisements and magazines as the gold standard. Many of those individuals are underweight. Instead, calculate the body mass index (BMI in kg/m^2) using height and body weight and the following formula:

BMI = weight in kg/square of the height in m

A healthy BMI is eighteen and a half to twenty-five. Some authors consider a value below twenty to be underweight. This is correct if this BMI is achieved through a highly restrictive pattern of eating. I do not consider it predictive of health-related problems if the individual is constitutionally of light build and weight has been stable for many years without any medical illness. A BMI between twenty-five (or twenty-seven) and thirty is overweight, between thirty and thirty-five is class one obesity, between thirty-five and forty, class two, and greater than forty, class three obesity.

Refer to the graph below to identify weight category using just the height and weight. The graph has been constructed using the former BMI categories. The values are in pounds, feet, and inches, since most of us are more comfortable with that system. The numerical values of the BMI will no longer be the same with these units. The same graph is used for men and women aged twenty to sixty-five years.

A significant limitation of the concept of BMI is that it does not account for weight gain in the form of muscle. In other words, the categories indicating health status are invalid if an individual is heavy for height because of muscle development. The BMI is useful for women in their childbearing years, that is, during the period leading to the onset of pregnancy. Women are at greater risk of developing complications if they are underweight or overweight at the beginning of their pregnancies. The BMI is not used during pregnancy.

Weight Categories Based on BMI

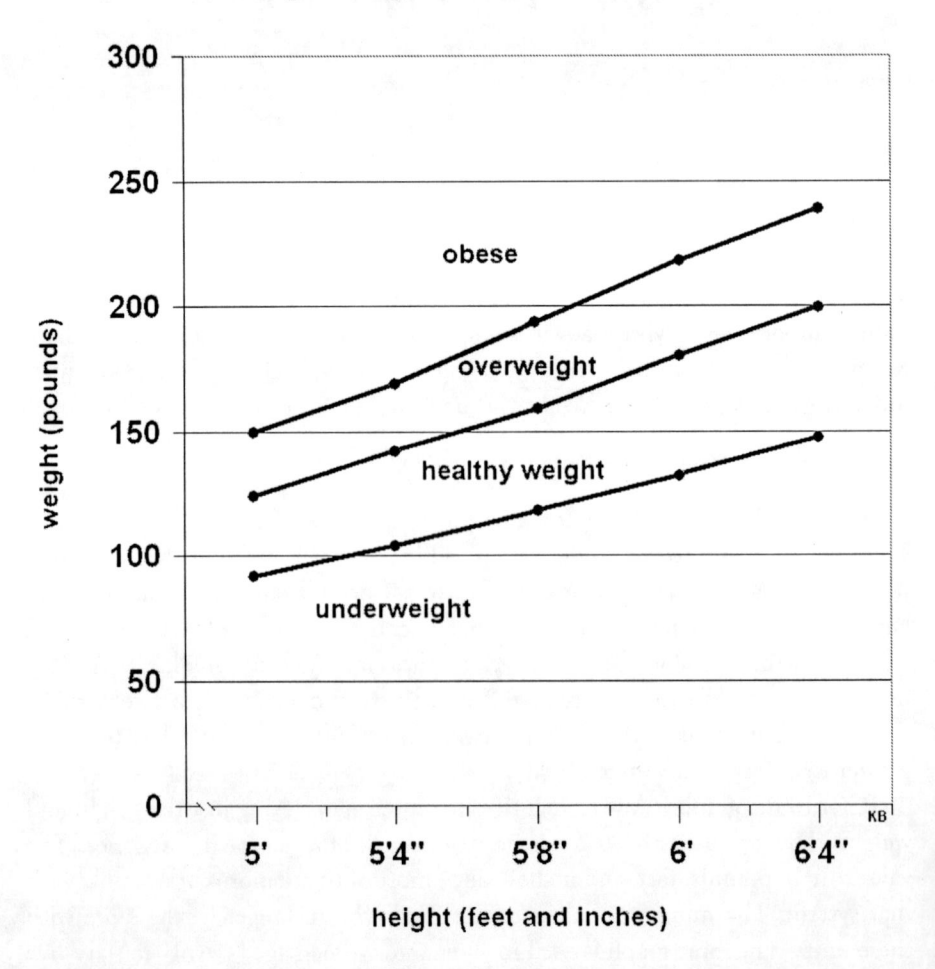

(Graph showing weight in pounds on the y-axis (0 to 300) versus height in feet and inches on the x-axis (5' to 6'4"), with curves delineating the categories: underweight, healthy weight, overweight, and obese.)

What are some of the other ways of looking at body weight? If body weight is double the ideal body weight or alternatively, one hundred pounds greater than ideal, then we use the term *morbid obesity*. One way to estimate desirable body weight in pounds is by using the following formulas:

> Adult male: 106 lb for the first 5 ft + 6 lb for every inch above
> Adult female: 105 lb for the first 5 ft + 5 lb for every inch above

If there is a preference for obtaining the results in kilograms, then the following formulas can be used:

Adult male: 50 kg for the first 5 ft + 2.3 kg for every inch above
Adult female: 45 kg for the first 5 ft + 2.3 kg for every inch above

However, the desirable body weight for an individual is not a discrete number but a range of weights. For this reason, BMI is a superior concept and now used more widely in doctors' offices. It encourages us to consider that a fairly large variation in body weight is compatible with good health.

WAIST SIZE

Another simple measurement that can be taken at home is waist size. If this is greater than forty inches (about 100 cm) in a man or thirty-six inches (90 cm) in a woman, then the risk of weight-related health problems rises significantly. This measurement is taken at the level of the umbilicus, or belly button, and not at the hips. The numbers will differ from pant waist size. These measurements are recorded upon arising in the morning or before consuming any meals, since food and drink will result in higher numbers. It is normal for meals to distend the belly, since all the internal and external structures in this part of the body are elastic.

Waist-to-hip ratios can also be calculated using these measurements. Ideally, this ratio should be less than 0.9 for men and less than 0.8 for women. Health risks are increased when this value is greater than 1.0 for both sexes. In other words, waist should be smaller than the hips.

Higher results will show that there is considerable fat tissue deposited around the middle or lower abdomen. This is referred to as *visceral obesity* in medicine and signals a particularly unhealthy form of weight deposition. It is commonly referred to as an "apple" body configuration. In contrast, others have a "pear" body type, in which fat is deposited on the lower body, i.e., the thighs, buttocks, and hips. This is *somatic obesity* and is usually associated with lower risk. Generally, men tend to develop apple shapes and women pear. Another way to look at this is that men carry their weight in front of themselves while women carry it behind!

OVERWEIGHT CHILDREN

Height and weight can be recorded and compared on standard growth charts, which are available at the doctor's office or on the Internet. Often, specific measurements are not really necessary to identify the overweight child, but they may be helpful if parents are not convinced. These children are typically the taller ones in schoolrooms. Their ultimate adult height is not necessarily greater than that of their leaner counterparts. This is because there is a significant individual variation in the rate of growth from child to child.

There is an abundance of fat deposited under the skin, with generous skin folds. Excessive enlargement of the breasts often proves embarrassing for boys. Genitals usually appear small because the base of the penis is embedded in fat in the pubic area. These factors do have a negative impact on body image and there may be reluctance to get involved in sports such as swimming, where some body exposure is required. A larger and heavier body frame sometimes proves beneficial in sports and social peer groups in youth. Moreover, heart disease and stroke are vague and remote problems as far as these kids are concerned. Overweight kids in this age group will need novel approaches and a lot of patience on the part of the family and the physician to ensure they do not grow into overweight adults.

The popular media as well as the medical profession tend to emphasize the problems that overweight children face in personal life and school. The perils of modern lifestyle choices are widely discussed. It is important to appreciate that the younger generation continues to attain greater height and stature along with higher intelligence quotients. Improved nutrition at critical times during growth is partly responsible for these results.

Children of immigrants pose further challenges for the health profession. These kids frequently reject traditional ethnic diets without having any appropriate alternate meal plan in place at home. The result is a dependence on commercial outlets and high-energy packaged snacks. Meanwhile, parents are often struggling to cope with a new environment and trying to meet basic financial goals. The resulting lack of time and discipline at home translates into a weight-control problem for their offspring.

BODY CONFIGURATION

It is often possible to classify body shapes into one of three types. Some individuals are tall and thin or have low body weight for their height. This is the *ectomor-*

phic body shape, which is commonly seen in basketball players. Others appear to have excessive weight for their height and may be described as overweight or chubby. This body type is called *endomorphic*. Finally, we find some individuals who appear muscular and stocky with little discernible fat tissue accounting for their size. These features are emphasized when they are short or medium in height, which gives an appearance of increased strength. This body shape is commonly found among football players. These individuals belong to the *mesomorphic* body type. When these individuals gain fat, they become larger and more formidable in appearance. This is the wrestler's build. Most of us fall somewhere in the middle of these extremes. I find this classification useful only when I am dealing with young adults, since aging, sedentary living, and weight gain change the shape of the body significantly.

RECOGNIZING DENIAL

The numbers may reinforce what the client already knows. Unfortunately, it is not always that straightforward. There are some individuals who refuse to acknowledge that they suffer from a weight problem; they are in *denial*. This is a defense mechanism that offers protection from unpleasant reality. Another common defense mechanism is *rationalization*, which is the justification of threatening feelings and behaviors through invalid explanations. Others realize that they have a weight problem but *have not made any commitment to do anything about it.* If somebody falls into any one of these categories, then their chances of success are going to be diminished.

These issues should be considered carefully before valuable time, money, and effort are invested in controlling weight. This is analogous to a nicotine or alcohol addiction. If the client does not make a commitment to do something about his or her problem, little will be accomplished. These endeavors require commitment on an indefinite basis in order to be successful.

When dealing with children, some parents fail to recognize that there is a problem in terms of weight or activity level. In such cases, it is useful to rely on the assessment performed by the physician and follow his or her advice. However, there should not be any confusion or diffusion of responsibility in this matter. The ultimate responsibility for children's lifestyle choices is borne by the parents.

ADVANTAGES OF BEING OVERWEIGHT

An informed decision should be made before deciding to lose weight. Are there any advantages to being heavy at any point in our lives? For example, physicians know that low body weight is associated with osteoporosis. The "middle-age spread" may confer some medical advantages by increasing mechanical stress on critical parts of our skeleton, such as the upper part of the thighbone located in our hip joints. A fracture in this part of our bodies may result in medical complications and may even result in death. It invariably requires a surgical operation for repair. Surgery carries not only the immediate risks associated with general anesthesia but also a number of potential post-operative complications, including pneumonia, heart failure, and so on. Hospitalization results in deconditioning. The patient may be left with a fear of falling.

The elderly frequently suffer from protein deficiency. Elderly males are at risk for inadequate nutritional and mineral reserves. Even the individual who has aged successfully may not have good nutritional reserves to cope with unforeseeable and inevitable medical problems. Those individuals who have lower body weight tend to have poorer outcomes in terms of survival at advancing age.

Reduced nutritional intake may be due to other factors, such as the lack of a spouse (where the senior no longer takes the effort to make good, quality meals). Other difficulties include cognitive impairment, poor eyesight, joint discomfort, chronic pain, chronic sadness, poor dentition, or a reduced ability to smell and taste food. There is also a reduction in appetite and absorption of many nutrients with advancing age. Individuals who are stooped due to a loss of height suffer from a "squashed stomach," which can result in a premature feeling of fullness. For reasons such as these, many health professionals are now recommending vitamin supplements for seniors. When BMI is related to mortality, we find that the lowest death rate for twenty to twenty-nine-year-olds is at a BMI close to twenty, whereas at ages sixty to sixty-nine years, it is at a BMI of twenty-seven. There is a natural tendency for BMI to decline after age sixty.

The problem is to age successfully without triggering a heart attack or cancer related to excessive weight. A good rule of thumb is that the younger the individual the more pressing is the importance of maintaining a healthy body weight. Most of us have come across news reports of serious weight-related problems in unusual age groups. We read about heart failure in children, heart attacks in young adults, and type II diabetes in teenagers. This type of diabetes is related to obesity in the majority of cases and was seen exclusively in middle-aged patients only a generation ago. Sedentary children also have poorer bone density, which will increase their risk of fractures throughout life. Obesity increases the risk of various forms of cancer, including large bowel, rectum, prostate, breast, ovaries, and uterus. Along with lung cancer, these malignancies account for most of the deaths attributed to cancer. There is also a higher incidence of gallbladder disease, which usually requires surgery for treatment.

Heavier patients undergoing surgery are at greater risk for complications. These include greater difficulty in maintaining blood oxygen levels, difficulty mobilizing, and prolonged recovery periods. These factors can interact and result in clots in the veins of the legs, a condition called *deep-vein thrombosis*. This is a particularly serious outcome since these clots can break off and travel to the lungs, interfering with both respiration and circulation. The workload of the heart is increased in this manner. Unfortunately, deep-vein thrombosis is a fairly challenging condition to diagnose. Studies have confirmed that physicians miss the diagnosis in a significant number of cases.

CASE HISTORY

RM, male
Age: 60 years
BMI: 26

I was a slight person in my youth, standing six feet tall and weighing 150 pounds. After nine months of police training, I put on thirty more pounds. My frame filled out with muscle. It was more difficult to maintain my weight after marriage, having a wonderful spouse who was a great cook. I was working at a detachment where the hours were long and the work very physical. I had a big appetite, but exercise kept my weight under control and my muscles well-toned. I took a position involving computers after twelve years. This entailed sitting for long periods. However, I also jogged, walked, skied, and swam. Even after twenty-two years at the desk job, my weight only went up to one hundred and eighty five pounds. I am now retired from the police force. We built a house ourselves near the ocean which involved landscaping as well. This was very hard work physically, but we took our time so as not to injure ourselves.

My hobbies now consist of golfing and building furniture. Golf is a great sport for the mind and body. I also try to walk two miles a day, although I am not able to do this each and every day. I have been able to maintain my weight within five pounds, although I know that I have lost muscle. I do have some arthritis in the knees, but otherwise my health is very good. I feel comfortable with my current body weight.

Breakfast consists of coffee, toast, and fruit. I have eggs once a week. I have a heart-healthy lunch consisting of carrots, turnips, cabbage, onions, and celery with a sandwich or crackers. We have a variety of vegetables and salad for dinner. We eat very little red meat, consuming chicken and fish for protein. We also try to avoid processed foods in general. I do enjoy desserts but make it a point to have these in moderation. Fruit is sometimes substituted for other desserts.

In my opinion, genes, moderation, and discipline have been the three factors that I consider most important in maintaining a healthy weight. I have had the good fortune of having a normal cholesterol and blood pressure. There are no serious medical problems so far. I try to eat and drink in moderation. My mother used to say, "Have a little bit of everything and you can have it all." Learn to say, "No, thank you" or "That is enough for now." It is difficult not to give in sometimes, but you will be glad that you held out later!

COMMENT

RM has maintained an excellent level of physical fitness through most of his adult life and has practiced healthy eating habits. Exercise appears to be an integral part of his lifestyle. Basically, he does not have to worry about weight gain. The BMI falls out of the healthy range because of muscle development and not fat. As discussed earlier, the BMI is appropriate due to age considerations.

2

Problems with Some Weight Control Strategies

COMMERCIAL PROGRAMS

A common question asked in doctors' offices is, "Should I join a weight loss program?" I want to stress again that a firm commitment is really the greatest component of the program. If a patient requires group sessions, peer support, and repeated counseling in order to obtain results, then he or she may not be able to *maintain* that loss when these props are not there. This is similar to the situation of the patient who tells the doctor: "Doc, I don't have any difficulty quitting smoking. I've done it dozens of times before!"

On a similar note, people will inquire about the safety or effectiveness of specific diets. A temporary weight loss can be expected from almost any form of regulation of one's dietary choices. There may be some information attesting to the "scientific" basis for these dietary programs. Unfortunately, the same individuals who are marketing these products often produce these writings. Medical doctors may not support these programs, since these so-called fad diets often lack a sound physiological basis. They may fail to gain acceptance by well-trained nutritional counselors. Some have obvious nutritional deficiencies and may be totally unsafe. Similarly, the long-term success of very low calorie diets has been attributed to ongoing counseling rather than the dramatic weight loss seen in the first few weeks.

Some of my patients have experienced significant weight reduction by restricting sugar and starches while increasing fat and protein intake. The presence of these carbohydrates in the blood is a key signal in our bodies to store energy. When sugars and starches are eliminated from the diet and the body's own stores are depleted, fat is mobilized rapidly. These changes have been called "metabolic starvation" because of some physiological similarities to starvation. The late Dr.

Atkins popularized this method of weight loss. Dietary supplements of micronutrients are part of the program since important foods, such as many fruits, have to be avoided.

This method was heavily criticized by the medical profession for many years and is still not approved generally. All the long-term consequences of a diet that is high in fat and protein are not known. Many physicians feel that they do not have an adequate understanding of the medical consequences, long-term success, and impact on life expectancy with this program. However, the consequences of neglecting a weight problem are well known. It is interesting that consumers have used this diet for decades without reports of serious medical consequences. A recent study confirmed that obese individuals lose more weight using a diet that is low in carbohydrates. Some patients have not been able to tolerate the diet reporting significant malaise. Others have failed to continue the program due to difficulty avoiding common food items such as bread, pasta, rice, potatoes, cookies, and pizza.

There are some dietary programs available that are based on current medically-recommended guidelines, which may be useful. If the client is unsure, he or she should collect as much literature as possible about the program and review it with a health professional. I do not approve of the use of many dietary supplements commonly found in supermarkets and health food stores. These preparations are meal substitutes that contain fewer calories. They are often expensive and really not necessary. One cannot stay on them to maintain results indefinitely anyway.

I feel that there should be a good understanding of human nutrition before significant changes in eating habits are made on any long-term basis. Most of us do not have the appropriate background or the time to invest in learning this subject. The key is to choose a sensible program that one can adhere to indefinitely. The emphasis should be on good nutrition and a healthy lifestyle. A program of this type should be available virtually free of charge. Many jurisdictions have authoritative guidelines available from public-health nurses, official health sites on the Internet, dietitians, and doctors' offices. These guidelines incorporate the best medical information into local norms. The more one tries to deviate from these guidelines, the greater will the likelihood be of failing to meet basic nutritional requirements. Similarly, a customized weight-loss program is going to be difficult to adhere to in the long run. It represents a short-term solution to a long-term problem. This will translate into a lack of weight control over the long term.

VEGETARIAN DIETS

We use the term *vegan* when the diet is strictly limited to foods of plant origin. Individuals who also consume milk products are *lactovegetarians* and those who accept eggs, *ovovegetarians*. Vegetarians who consume milk and eggs are lactovovegetarians. Vegans risk deficiencies in essential amino acids, calcium, zinc, iron, as well as vitamins D and B12. Many of these difficulties can be resolved with the addition of eggs and milk into the diet or by the use of supplements. Let us examine some of these issues further.

Adolescents will sometimes adopt this lifestyle as an assertion of their individualism. However, this age group is at high risk of failing to meet nutritional requirements. The vegan diet may be deficient in fat, so that they may fail to meet their energy requirements. Protein will be used for energy during a period when it is required for growth. Moreover, there are eight amino acids that the body cannot make. These are referred to as *essential amino acids*. These are readily obtained in food derived from animal sources. A lack of these protein building blocks will interfere with the efficient use of available protein and affect growth and development. Therefore, the daily protein requirement for vegans is fifty percent higher than that of individuals on a mixed diet. Strength athletes who are meat consumers can easily meet their protein requirements without supplements, whereas this will be difficult for vegans.

Dietary calcium and iron are absorbed efficiently from animal sources. Avoidance of meat and fish may result in poor iron reserves. The consumption of tea with meals will impair iron uptake further. This is due partly to the presence of a group of chemicals found in tea called *tannins*. A high intake of fiber is known to interfere with iron absorption as well. This is due to the presence of another group of chemicals in fiber-rich food, known as *phytates*. However, some researchers have shown that the incidence of iron deficiency is no greater among vegetarians than those consuming a mixed diet. A number of other factors are clearly involved.

A vegan diet is frequently high in vitamin C, which markedly increases the absorption of iron from plant sources. Vitamin C is found in citrus fruit, fortified fruit juices, tomatoes, and green leafy vegetables. An interesting observation is that the iron content of plant-derived food is actually higher than that of meat sources in many cases when the amount of iron is related to the energy derived from that same food. In this manner, a well-planned vegan diet is compatible with adequate iron reserves.

Iron stores can last three years in men, whereas women only have enough for three months on the North American meat-based diet. Iron deficiency is associated with a low blood level, a condition called *anemia*. Iron is associated with hemoglobin, which is the protein involved with the transport of oxygen in blood. Hemoglobin is carried in red blood cells, giving blood its red color. When the body is deficient in iron, the production of these cells is impaired, eventually leading to anemia and reduced oxygen-carrying capacity. The symptoms of this condition include pallor, fatigue, shortness of breath with exertion, and dizziness. Dizziness is more noticeable when changing position, for example, arising from a lying position. Iron deficiency is the most common nutrient deficiency. High-risk groups include infants, adolescent girls, and women in their reproductive years and during pregnancy. Women have especially high requirements for iron due to the monthly loss of blood in menstrual cycles. It is common practice to prescribe iron supplements in pregnancy.

Iron deficiency is also found in seniors who live on a poor "tea and toast" diet. However, iron deficiency can also result from increased losses from the body. Therefore, these patients are often investigated for peptic ulcers and bowel cancer. Meat and vegetarian sources of iron are listed below.

Pork and beef	Lentils
Liver, kidney, heart	Prune juice
Clams, oysters	Soy flour
Baked beans, lima beans, kidney beans	Almonds
Peas, pea soup, chickpeas	
Dried fruit, such as apricot, prunes, figs, and raisins	

The increased fiber content in vegetarian meals has been found to interfere with zinc absorption as well. Zinc is a crucial mineral for growth and tissue repair. Inadequate zinc levels have been identified in American seniors and adolescent girls on mixed diets. Mild deficiency can cause growth impairment in children. It is also vital for proper functioning of the reproductive system. Good sources of zinc are listed below:

Beef and Pork	Lentils
Oysters and crab	Nuts
Poultry	Peas

Egg yolk	Bran
Milk	Dried beans

Calcium intake is a controversial topic among health professionals. We have seen significant changes to the medical recommendations for daily intakes of this mineral recently. These values have been increased. In contrast, the values are lower in other countries. It has been suggested that the North American diet, which is high in protein derived from meat and dairy products, actually increases calcium loss in the urine. This has resulted in increased requirements of this mineral. The vegan diet has lower amounts of protein and the calcium requirements may also be lower. Certain plant-derived foods are high in *oxalic acid* and are not considered good sources of calcium, since this substance interferes with absorption. Spinach, beet greens, tea, and almonds are examples of foods that have oxalic acid. Similarly, high-fiber foods containing phytate also reduce calcium absorption.

Information on the impact of different dietary habits upon bone mineralization is starting to appear now that measurements of bone density are becoming more widespread. A study performed on Chinese subjects showed lower hip-bone densities in vegans compared to those on mixed diets. A list of calcium-rich foods derived from animal and plant sources is provided below.

Milk, yogurt, and cheese	Mustard greens
Sardines with bones	Collards
Turnip greens, turnip	Soybeans and tofu
Legumes	Oranges, tangerines
Broccoli	Dried fruit (dates, figs, prunes, raisins)
Kale	Almonds

Vitamin B12 is needed in very small amounts for the production of blood cells and for the proper functioning of the brain, spinal cord, and peripheral nerves. It is available only in foods of animal origin but can be found in fortified cereals and other select vegetarian foods. Liver stores of this vitamin last a decade or more, so a deficiency takes a long time to develop in vegans who had been consuming a mixed diet.

Vitamin B12 deficiency is not uncommon in the elderly, largely due to a loss in the ability to absorb this chemical. Stomach acidity helps to release this vitamin from ingested food. There may be reduction in stomach acid production with age or due to the use of powerful inhibitors found in prescription medications. Some individuals lose the chemical machinery, found in the wall of the stomach, designed to absorb vitamin B12. The physician may first suspect a deficient state based on the shape of the blood cells. These cells have a high requirement of this vitamin and will often become visibly abnormal. Frank anemia, known as *pernicious anemia*, may develop. In some cases, the blood may continue to appear normal but the patient will exhibit psychiatric symptoms or complain of abnormal sensations in the arms or legs. These changes are not always reversible when the diagnosis is established and the vitamin is replaced. Vegans will have to make a special effort to ensure that they are consuming appropriate amounts of this vitamin.

Although vegetarianism is considered a food fad in North America, it is the norm in some parts of the world. Unfortunately, many of those individuals also lack access to appropriate dietary counseling, resulting in widespread deficiencies in basic nutrients and minerals and preventing them from reaching their full genetic potential. In this manner, iron deficiency is commonplace in children and adults in many parts of the world. This mineral has been shown to play an important role in the cognitive development of children. In developing countries, anemia resulting from iron deficiency is a leading cause of death in women at the time of childbirth, when there is further blood loss. Anemia joins malnutrition and infection as the three most common causes of morbidity and mortality in many areas of the world. These deficiencies are largely avoidable through appropriate education and inexpensive supplements.

Vegetarianism does not result in a lower intake of fat or reduce the risk of heart disease when poor food choices are made on a repeated basis. Breads are frequently covered with butter or margarine before consumption, increasing energy values. Vegetables that are deep-fried or served with fatty dips or butter are no longer lean servings. Similarly, excessive consumption of foods such as fruit can aggravate weight gain by providing another source of calories. A carefully planned vegetarian diet can be a useful way to control weight since these diets generally have lower energy values compared to mixed diets. Medical researchers have shown significant reductions in recurrent heart disease in heart patients consuming a low-fat vegetarian diet.

This dietary pattern does prevent *constipation*, although many individuals complain of bloating. It is also associated with a lower incidence of *appendicitis*, *diverticulosis*, and cancer of the large bowel. The reduction in bowel cancer has been attributed to the elimination of red meat from the diet along with the presence of fiber. A dietary consultation is recommended if a vegetarian lifestyle is being considered during childhood, adolescence, pregnancy, breastfeeding, or the senior years.

WEIGHT CYCLING

A significant public-health issue called weight cycling has been identified. This refers to a pattern of relatively rapid weight loss followed by a tendency to regain all of the weight within twelve to twenty-four months. This leads to frustration followed by a renewal of one's determination, and the cycle begins again. It is suspected that this pattern leads to a number of adverse medical conditions. It may accelerate bone calcium loss and promote osteoporosis, although a recent research article could not substantiate this.

A culturally appropriate program compatible with family background as well as personal preferences should be chosen. The patterns that should be established *have to be life-long*. If this is not accomplished, the chances of failure in the long run are going to be high. Many obese individuals can tolerate losing four or five pounds monthly for prolonged periods. Rapid weight reduction is not necessary; the goal should be sustained results.

ANOREXIA AND BULIMIA

A healthy desire to maintain a normal body weight should be distinguished from abnormal behaviors. A weight loss achieved by self-induced vomiting, strict dietary regimens, use of laxatives, dehydration, and hyper-exercising are not compatible with good health.

Is it possible that the individual has a distorted picture of how he or she should look? The following inquiries can be made in addition to uncovering some of the abnormal behaviors listed above: Have you chosen to be a fashion model, a dancer, or a gymnast? Have you ever felt weak and dizzy or fainted when restricting your eating? Are you pale and tired, and have your monthly menstrual cycles stopped? If the answer is yes to any of these questions, an honest discussion should be held with a physician. These can be symptoms of a serious medical condition called *anorexia nervosa*.

Bulimia refers to repeated cycles of weight gain through uncontrollable eating followed by weight loss through vomiting. These are two types of eating disorders that appear to be coping mechanisms to deal with inner problems that are too difficult to address directly. These conditions will require frequent visits to health professionals so that serious trends can be identified. These disorders are primarily seen in adolescent girls and younger women. Many others report a preoccupation with body image and may adopt a very restricted pattern of eating. Thus, meals may be consumed irregularly and certain food groups may be avoided.

Young men may also have a distorted image of their bodies due to heavy influence by peer pressure, magazines, and advertising. They may spend excessive time trying to develop muscle and take supplements, including banned male hormones, in order to achieve this goal. When these activities become distressing and uncontrollable, interfering with normal day-to-day life, professionals use the term *body dysmorphic disorder*.

CASE HISTORY

GM, male
Age: 58 years
BMI: 43, now 35

I have struggled with weight problems for many years. I did not participate in any sports or exercise program all my adult life. My usual diet had a number of rich foods including meat, milk, eggs, cheese, and snack foods as well. I always ate three meals a day. My breakfast would usually consist of fried eggs, bacon or ham, and toast. I worked in an office at a desk job for most of my career and I probably did not need to eat as much as I did. Fortunately, I did not smoke or drink.

Several members of my family are overweight. Some went on to develop problems with blood pressure and diabetes in mid-life. My doctor is treating me for high blood pressure and thyroid problems with medications. My cholesterol has always been good. I do not suffer from diabetes.

I have tried many different diets over the years but was never able to stay with them for any length of time. I found that I did not like the food that was on the diet sheet or that I was hungry. A friend told me about the Atkins diet and I purchased one of the books dealing with it. I started the diet in February of last year at a weight of 290 pounds. I found the concepts in the diet appealing, as I had always been a high-protein consumer.

I lost fifteen pounds in the first two weeks. I felt much better with a lot more energy. I find that my energy level is increasing as I continue to lose more weight.

I am able to do things that were difficult before. I find the diet quite easy to follow and I am seldom hungry. I have to monitor the ketone levels in urine. I keep these at "trace" levels. The amount of food that a person can eat does not seem as important as it does with other diets, no more measuring or weighing food. Remember, watch the carbohydrates. For example my wife, who does most of the cooking, has recipes that remove white flour from bread. Now, my bread has rolled oats, soy flour, and wheat gluten.

I feel there has to be a lifelong commitment to maintain the weight loss with this diet. I do not think that it is going to be difficult for me to do this. I lost forty pounds in the first six months. I have not lost much more since, but I am very happy with the results.

COMMENT

I have been working with GM for many years now. He did not make any progress with our discussions regarding lifestyle issues. Perhaps what he learned was that he had to do something about his severe weight problem. I am pleased to see that he has accomplished some of the goals that we wanted. I find that patients who are achieving results with Dr. Aitkins' diet report that hunger is not an obstacle. I appreciate that these patients feel well and exhibit a sense of empowerment.

Dr. Atkins' diet is based on well-known physiology. The diet induces a state of fat breakdown using hormonal mechanisms. I have worked with hospitalized patients who were placed on very low calorie diets, with daily blood monitoring, to achieve weight reduction. This approach is avoidable since we can achieve the same state using Dr. Atkins' method. Unfortunately, there is a lot of controversy surrounding the Atkins approach. I believe that this is largely unnecessary. Traditionally, physicians learn about the best dietary principles in the ideal individual. Application of these principles to individuals with severe difficulties with appetite may not be realistic.

There is production of ketones by the elimination of simple carbohydrates in the initial phase of the diet. This should not be confused with the dangerous metabolic changes found in uncontrolled, type I diabetes (see chapter seven). We do not have a complete understanding of the long-term safety of this diet. However, I do not discourage patients from achieving their goals using this approach because there is ample evidence of the risks associated with obesity. I have not found evidence in the medical literature of serious risks with the Atkins method.

3

Getting Started

RULING OUT PHYSICAL PROBLEMS

Medical problems should be ruled out at the beginning of any attempt to regulate weight. There are many physical grounds for excessive weight, which can be determined through a check of the patient's medical and family history and a physical examination, performed by a physician. Genetic disorders may be responsible, but hormonal problems are much more common.

An important finding may be a personal or family history of *hypothyroidism*. In this disorder, the *thyroid gland,* which is located just below the voice box, functions at a reduced level, producing lower levels of the hormone *thyroxine*. This will result in a lower metabolic rate and result in symptoms such as weight gain, cold intolerance, constipation, excessive sleepiness, and dry skin. The full constellation of symptoms occurs fairly late in the course of this disorder and the diagnosis may be missed. Instead, the problem can be detected readily through blood tests that measure *thyroid-stimulating hormone* and thyroxine. Hypothyroidism is classified as an autoimmune disorder whereby the body's own immune system targets a specific tissue, leading to derangement of structure and function. Disorders of this type are more prevalent in women.

Another problem that physicians can assess includes *Cushing's disease,* in which fat distributes on the torso, resulting in *truncal obesity*. There may also be an elevation in blood pressure and thinning of the skin with this disorder. A diagnosis that can be considered in female patients is called *polycystic ovarian disease*. In its classical form, this disorder results in obesity, hirsutism (excessive body hair in inappropriate locations), and menstrual irregularities. We believe that polycystic ovarian disease is triggered by excessive body weight and that weight loss is an important consideration in treatment.

Weight gain is often discussed in the context of *depression*. Depression is frequently associated with derangements of vegetative functions, such as sleeping and appetite. The symptoms of this disorder include pervasive sadness, loss of enjoyment in many activities that were formerly pleasurable, fatigue, diminished concentration, early awakenings, and reduced libido. Some individuals experience an increase in appetite while others lose interest in food. Often, there is a positive family history of this disorder, especially on the maternal side. There may be precipitating events as well.

When dealing with this clinical situation, my approach is to address the underlying problem, which is the mood disorder, namely depression, and hope that the appetite will regulate itself. This also implies that I do not consider weight gain to be an important factor in triggering clinical depression, in most cases. The common clinical scenario is that we, as physicians, focus on the treatment of depression and struggle with the patient to make them feel better. The weight that has been gained assumes secondary importance, and it is seldom lost. The finding that some of the medications that are used to treat depression are associated with weight gain compounds the problem.

Many others do not have all the symptoms of a major mood disorder, yet suffer from chronic unhappiness, a condition called *dysthymia*. An inability to maintain a healthy body weight may be aggravated by this condition. The physician will need to explore the patient's overall life situation in order to achieve progress. The patient may not appreciate the physical impact of a stressful job or an unhappy marriage.

Many patients suffer from a peculiar lack of sleep quality that health-care professionals call *obstructive sleep apnea*. This is almost exclusively observed in very overweight individuals. Part of the explanation for this is the extra mass of tissue found around the upper airway. This tissue collapses around the airway during sleep-induced relaxation. In this disorder, the individual often snores loudly and has periods where he or she stops moving air into the lungs, a period known as *apnea*. They cannot volunteer this information because they are essentially asleep during these events.

When these individuals are monitored in sleep laboratories, they are found to desaturate; that is, the oxygen level declines. These individuals will awaken to restore breathing hundreds of times during the night without being aware that they are doing this. They are also vulnerable to heart attacks during those periods of oxygen desaturation. These individuals will experience fatigue and easy sleeping, or *hypersomnolence*, during the daytime.

As we have seen, heavier individuals are much more prone to obstructive sleep apnea because of the weight of the soft tissues around the throat. This problem is aggravated by sedatives, including alcohol. Alcohol results in an abnormal pattern of sleep with further relaxation of the soft tissues of the neck, increasing snoring and obstructive breathing patterns. Similarly, sleeping pills that are called *hypnotics* are inappropriate for these individuals when attempting to restore restful sleep.

The body's primitive defense mechanisms to cope with fatigue start to operate. The body reacts by building energy stores and chronic hunger and overeating are triggered. Weight climbs and the cycle just goes on until the problem is identified and addressed. This syndrome is particularly prevalent in older, overweight men. However, it remains undiagnosed in over eighty percent of cases. Sometimes, physicians will prescribe weight loss as first line of treatment. The alternatives are more invasive and may even involve surgery. When both the underlying weight problem and the nighttime breathing disorder remain uncontrolled, heart failure can result. The full disorder—with obesity, abnormal nighttime breathing, daytime sleepiness, and heart failure—is called the *Pickwickian syndrome*.

Obstructive sleep apnea is not limited to adults. Children can have obstructive breathing due to enlarged adenoids and tonsils and may experience the same fatigue. They may demonstrate irritability and school failure as a result of this problem.

Overweight individuals also suffer from breathing difficulties resulting from an impaired ability of the chest to expand. This is a mechanical problem resulting from the excessive weight of the chest wall and the inability of the diaphragm to push down. This is called *restrictive lung disease of obesity*. This is associated with lower oxygen levels in blood as well.

It is advisable to consider that a portion of the extra body weight is fluid. As a rule, rapid changes in body weight are due to fluid loss or gain. This may be a sign of a serious underlying disorder such as kidney disease, congestive heart failure, or liver disease. The fluid may be in the dependent parts of the body, such as the ankles, in which case it is called *peripheral edema*. If it is in the abdomen, it is called *ascitis*. *Pulmonary edema* is the presence of fluid in the lung air spaces and is an especially dangerous sign. The individual with pulmonary edema will become short of breath when lying down and may have resorted to propping, using more and more pillows. A physician can rule out all these disorders. When the patient suffers from any of these problems, body weight can be recorded on a regular basis weekly or biweekly and presented at clinical visits.

THE PHYSICIAN'S ROLE

The client should work closely with knowledgeable health professionals, including physicians and dietitians. These individuals have a considerable amount of training and expertise in these matters. These issues have come to the forefront of modern medicine in recent decades. We now believe that preventative medicine is an important component in the delivery of medical care. Family doctors are no longer solely dedicated to the treatment of disease but would like to see patients take the necessary steps to prevent problems from developing. Accordingly, an essential component in a successful weight-control program is the commitment of the patient. There is virtually no limit to what motivated individuals can do to address lifestyle issues once they have obtained the appropriate medical information.

CASE HISTORY

JS, male
Age: 33 years
BMI: initially 40, now 35

I am a thirty-three old male. For two years, I worked in an environment that was personally very stressful. At that time, I was easily fatigued and I experienced a sense of malaise. I consulted a physician who diagnosed depression and prescribed an antidepressant. It was suggested in these consultations that I make some lifestyle changes with respect to diet and physical activity, which are often helpful in dealing with stress and depression.

I took this advice into consideration and did a self-assessment of my lifestyle. I used published medical food guides as the objective standard to which I would compare my present diet. I concluded that my diet was lacking in variety and not appropriate in several ways. Physical activity was almost nonexistent in my life. I then decided to make some changes.

I began by following food guides and eating the recommended types and variety of foods. However, I deviate from the guide one day a week and indulge in my favorite "junk foods." I also started to walk three kilometers five days a week. I increased the distance to five kilometers after three months. About three months later, I started to alternate between walking and jogging. I measured out a distance of one kilometer and I would walk from one utility pole to the next;

then I would jog from that pole to the next until the kilometer was completed. Nowadays, my main aerobic exercise is jogging, although I walk occasionally. I jog two and a half kilometers in twenty minutes. A few months into the walking routine, I introduced strength training. I now lift weights three times a week.

Eight months later, I feel that I have benefited greatly from these lifestyle changes physically. I have lost thirty-one pounds and no longer fatigue easily. The malaise has also disappeared completely. I have noticed a significant improvement in my mental and emotional health. I have a greater capacity to handle stress and to concentrate. Of course, some of these improvements can be attributed to the antidepressant. However, I did take antidepressants in the past without making any changes in lifestyle and the results were only marginal.

COMMENT

This individual was highly motivated in spite of a mood disorder and demonstrated significant weight loss through well-established medical principles. He discovered that he had been making unhealthy food choices previously. He also had a sedentary lifestyle.

4

Energy Balance

THE CALORIE

An understanding of the concept of energy balance should be developed early in any discussion of weight control. The *calorie* is a measure of the energy available from food substances or expended during the performance of a task (also see glossary). Body weight remains stable when the amount of energy derived from ingested food equals the amount used up for autonomic body functions and physical effort.

      Energy consumed = energy expended

If more calories are consumed than used up, or "burned," there is a *positive caloric balance* and the excess nutrition is deposited in the form of fat. Hence, the individual will gain body mass and weight. Conversely, more energy needs to be spent than consumed in order to mobilize fat, that is, to achieve a *negative calorie balance*.

This powerful concept explains issues patients sometimes find confusing. They will often complain that they cannot lose weight even though they appear to eat very little compared to others around them. They say that the hardest thing about dieting isn't watching what you eat but watching what others eat! These individuals have reached a plateau with a new set point in body weight. They still need to turn things around and tip the equation, that is, increase energy expenditure.

USING THE ENERGY EQUATION

Looking again at the equation above, you will see a fairly straightforward approach to weight control. It is this: one can get results by reducing the left side of the equation, that is, by lowering the amount of calories ingested. The activity level does not have to change. This is useful in many individuals who are physically less capable of exercise, such as those who are wheelchair-dependent. Similarly, if one already suffers from chronic pain in the knees, as many overweight people do, they are not in a position to start jogging or high-impact aerobics. The elderly, who may have suffered coronary events or strokes already, can also take advantage of this relationship.

Clients must have a complete appreciation of these concepts before they are going to see results. It should also reinforce the idea that they should not be paying more to get less. This is how some expensive dietary programs work. They pay to consume a preparation with a fancy label that provides fewer calories. Instead, they can lower energy consumption in their daily meals.

DAILY ENERGY REQUIREMENTS

If the client would like to count calories, an estimate of the maintenance requirements can be calculated easily. The number of calories that an active adult male needs in a twenty-four-hour period (Calories/day) is determined by his ideal body weight in kilograms (one kilogram is equal to 2.2 pounds) multiplied by thirty-five. The corresponding figure for an active adult woman is thirty. Reduce or increase these figures by five if the individual is sedentary or *very* active respectively. For example, a woman weighing sixty kilograms who is very active requires (60 kg x 35) 2,100 Calories/day. These figures result in approximate energy requirements of 1,800–2,000 Calories for women and 2,000–2,500 for men.

Reduce daily requirements by ten percent for each decade past age fifty due to a lower basal metabolic rate and level of activity.

To calculate the approximate number of calories one needs to consume in order to *lose* body weight, multiply the ideal body weight by twenty. For example, if ideal weight is eighty kilograms, then daily caloric intake will have to be reduced to about (80 x 20) 1,600 Calories/day. Remember that one should not consume less than 1,200 Calories/day if a woman or 1,500 Calories/day if a man in order to meet minimum nutritional requirements. In more practical terms, a daily reduction of 500 Calories from the meal plan will result in a four-pound weight loss monthly. This is a realistic goal for most people.

Approximations of this type are available for children as well. Allow one thousand Calories for the first year of life, then one hundred Calories for each subsequent year of life. Let us look at an example. An eight-year-old child will need

(1,000 + (100 x 7)) 1,700 Calories/day. Obviously, children have special nutritional needs, and a qualified dietitian must be involved in any significant long-term modifications in eating habits.

CALORIES IN FAST FOOD

If you find these numbers interesting, then also examine the calorie content of food items. These lists are readily available on the Internet or through the office of a dietitian. I will not reproduce them here, but let us consider some examples to address the issue of fast food.

	Calories	fat (g)
Commercial hamburger with cheese	550	30
French fries, medium	300	15
Milk shake	300	12
Pepperoni pizza, personal size	675	30
Chicken sandwich	480	25
Cole slaw	120	7

Note: All values are approximate.

If Tom decided to avoid cooking a meal and went into the local fast food outlet for an order of a hamburger, French fries, and a milk shake, he would consume 1,150 Calories and fifty-seven grams of fat. Let us assume that his daily total caloric requirements were 2,400 Calories. He would have met almost one half of the day's energy requirements in one meal. Recommended daily fat consumption is sixty grams for women and ninety grams for men. A woman would have consumed the entire day's recommended fat intake in one sitting! Since there are nine Calories derived from a gram of fat, 513 of the 1,150 Calories, or forty-five percent of the calories in this meal, are from fat. Generally, forty to sixty percent of calories from fast foods are derived from fat. Guidelines recommend that calories derived from fat should not exceed thirty percent. Other poor fast food choices are donuts and poutine. Chicken and fish items at fast-food outlets are also quite fatty since they are usually coated in batter and deep-fried.

It is not unusual nowadays for younger members of society to visit a convenient fast-food location for a 9:00 p.m. "snack" a few times a week. A relatively small change in behavior will have a tremendous benefit in terms of the overall energy intake.

FOOD RECORDS

If the patient is not interested in counting calories, an excellent way to develop familiarity with these concepts is the three-day food record. This requires that the individual write down the food item and the quantity consumed over an average three-day period. One should not rely on memory but make a prospective list of all the items that are eaten or drank. Accuracy and honesty are important when doing this. It would be helpful to provide details in the margins, such as whether cream or milk was used in coffee or the type of fat that was used to fry the breakfast egg. This list is then taken to the physician, or better still to the dietitian, for review. These health-care workers can calculate the total number of calories consumed on a daily basis and point out drawbacks in some of the choices, followed by suggestions.

The qualitative aspect of this information will quickly improve one's understanding of nutrition. Incidentally, computer programs are now available that can generate these types of data. However, the client might learn more by dealing with a health-care worker.

NUTRITION AND WEIGHT

Consider blood tests after a weight problem has been identified. Unfortunately, the consumption of a large amount of calories does not remedy nutritional deficiencies in all cases. It is not uncommon to discover that overweight teenage girls suffer from deficient iron stores. Many others consume insufficient amounts of folic acid, other B vitamins, vitamin C, calcium, zinc, and vitamin D. These nutritional deficiencies may be aggravated by attempts at calorie restriction. A professional will be able to identify problems of this nature and show that the new diet will also have more essential vitamins, amino acids, and calcium.

Some overweight clients show signs of excessive insulin secretion even though they do not have diabetes. These signs include fluid retention in the feet and ankles, visceral obesity, high blood pressure, abnormal lipid profiles (called *dyslipidemias*), and *atherosclerosis*, or fat deposition in blood vessels. Important blood tests include fasting sugar (or glucose) levels and fasting lipids.

It is important to appreciate that normal serum calcium values are not helpful in quantifying the intake of this mineral. Similarly, these numbers provide little information regarding the complex physiological changes that occur when the body regulates blood calcium levels. Chronic nutritional deficiency of this mineral will result in an increase in a hormone called the *parathyroid hormone*, which reabsorbs calcium from bones. Eventually, this will result in the devastating loss of bone strength found in osteoporosis. Similarly, a blood test is not readily available to determine vitamin D levels. A good dietary history and food records remain vital sources of information in this area.

Some individuals make the mistake of assuming all is well because they feel well. Unfortunately, many of these problems can be clinically silent, especially in the early stages. These include serious disorders such as high blood pressure, diabetes, atherosclerosis, lipid abnormalities, and bone loss. Similarly, children can suffer from some of the same disorders that we previously associated with lifestyle or degenerative problems. Physicians do not have clear guidelines based on research regarding screening in children. The physician will individualize these recommendations until such data are available.

CASE HISTORY

BP, female
Age: 41 years
BMI: 42

I had been told for as long as I can remember that my family had a healthy appetite. Many family members were all overweight, and that was not considered a bad thing. I recall descriptions such as "He is solid" applied to some of my relatives. According to my earliest recollection, my own weight problem began in my late teens, when my appetite suddenly blossomed. I developed poor eating habits in high school and during post-secondary education. I remember snacking on quickly-prepared foods while studying.

My first full-time job involved working shifts, which led to irregular eating habits. At home, I was cooking large meals, since my husband was a laborer performing strenuous physical activity. My appetite was fair during the first few months I was pregnant with my first child. However, it increased tremendously later on, and I felt that there was no need to try and control it, since I was eating for two. It remained very good while I was breast-feeding my nine-pound, four-ounce baby boy. He required frequent feedings that left no time for any physical activity outdoors. My second pregnancy began ten months after delivery. Soon the stress of full-time shift work, a husband working away from home, and leaving my babies in someone else's care were taking a toll. Food provided some emotional satisfaction and turned out to be a great coping mechanism. Then came my third pregnancy. In that crucial year, my husband also suffered a work-related injury that required surgery. He was disabled for several months. The stress was also aggravated by the death of a close relative and the fact that my oldest child was starting school. I was taking care of three kids as well as helping my husband try to get back to a job that was very demanding physically. It was apparent that he would not be able to return to that job as time passed.

I returned to school to further my education, provide myself with some intellectual challenge, and get away from shift work. The toll on the mind, body, and spirit were intense. Poor eating habits became a mechanism for coping. It was ironic that the very study of preventive health promotion was forcing me to ignore my own health and well-being. There were huge demands on my time, leaving little for me. I experienced frequent minor illnesses, insomnia, and fatigue as a busy mother, wife, primary wage earner, and student. Food became a solace, and there was little time to plan or cook healthy meals. I opted for the eat-on-the-run types of foods that were easy to prepare.

I come from a very close-knit family. A woman's worth was often determined by her cooking skills. These meals were often very rich and included a lot of desserts and baked pastries. Social gatherings in the family, community, or church also centered on large meals. A large appetite was admired and others were labeled picky eaters. I have lost weight using commercial dietary programs only to regain what I had lost, and then some. I keep saying that I will worry about myself tomorrow, when things are less hectic. Right now, others are more important to me. It is also difficult to cook for growing kids while preparing a separate low-calorie item for myself. I am just trying to keep a busy household going while maintaining a demanding and stressful career.

It is hard to blame any one factor for my weight problem. It is a complicated mixture of heredity, habits, emotions, environment, and life circumstances. It is an ongoing struggle. Even though I am fully qualified to teach others about the importance of good nutrition and exercise, I have difficulty setting a good example.

COMMENT

This is the story of a bright woman who has a successful career. She has managed to raise a lovely family as well. Unfortunately, we have failed to control her problem with body weight. Her BMI is in the obese category and she risks many of the problems discussed in this book, including osteoarthritis, hypertension, diabetes, premature heart disease, cancer, and early mortality. She is on medications for high blood pressure already. She declined to use medications for controlling her weight.

5

Physical Activity

ENERGY EXPENDITURE

Recalling the energy balance equation, we can understand how regular physical activity can promote weight loss. I am going to explore this issue in detail later but you might want to study some numbers first in order to appreciate this concept. Again, tables are available on the Internet and elsewhere. An individual weighing 150 pounds uses eighty to ninety Calories per hour sitting and resting. Energy expenditure increases threefold with housework, fourfold walking, fivefold swimming or cycling, and tenfold with competitive games such as squash, soccer, or tennis. Climbing stairs utilizes about six hundred Calories hourly.

It is clear that a sedentary lifestyle is a key factor in many individuals suffering from weight gain. Couple this with long hours of watching television and energy expenditure declines further due to the reduction in spontaneous activity.

ACTIVE LIFESTYLE

I have mentioned stair-climbing, walking, and housework for good reasons. Expensive memberships to fitness centers are not always necessary; their main feature is that they enable us to adhere to a routine once a monetary commitment has been made. Perhaps the most significant factor in the ubiquitous increase in body fat seen in affluent societies is a reduction in hour-to-hour energy utilization. We drive to work, use elevators, sit at desk jobs, use automated car washes, use washing machines, and hire kids to mow our lawns.

Performing everyday tasks around the home can use up a significant amount of calories and energy. Examples include walking around the neighborhood, walking the dog, housework, gardening, mowing, and washing the car. These activities can be spontaneous, depending on occupational duties and lifestyle;

however, the benefits appear mainly when performed regularly and frequently. Making a more vigorous effort can increase energy expenditure. Let us examine climbing stairs. If there is a multistory home, there are benefits just walking upstairs several times a day. This is part of the reason behind seniors abandoning five-bedroom mansions for condominiums. It takes a significant amount of effort, not to mention good health, to maintain these homes. Clearly, these are things that can be incorporated into the daily routine on a long-term basis.

The concepts discussed above may become clearer when quantified. Measurements show that a pound (or 454 g) of fat tissue yields approximately 3,500 Calories of energy. Suppose we were to incorporate a fifteen-minute walk into the daily routine or perform fifteen minutes of housework on a daily basis. This would use sixty or more Calories each day and account for a *thirty-pound weight loss* over five years. In this way, multiple changes in lifestyle that may each appear trivial can help prevent weight gain or result in a successful loss of weight for others.

Not too long ago, a retiree complained to me about the hard work she had to do at home on a daily basis while her husband led a sedentary lifestyle. I noted that she looked fit and trim while he had the usual apple configuration and was looking at a coronary bypass in the not-too-distant future. I am not sure for whom I actually felt sorry. The take home message: share in the household chores and both of you can reap the benefits. Get that walk-behind mower out more often and make your lawn the envy of the neighborhood!

A major exception in the list of daily tasks is the shoveling of snow. This activity is inadvisable after age thirty-five years unless one has maintained a high level of fitness. Studies have shown that a significant isometric effort is required to lift a shovel loaded with snow, which is associated with a rapid rise in heart rate. At the same time, there are multiple changes in blood flow to different parts of the body. Blood vessels in the skin are narrowed or constricted in cold ambient temperatures while those to exercising muscles are dilated or expanded. The vessels supplying the heart may narrow in response to cold exposure as well. Many individuals have already developed significant but asymptomatic narrowing in one or more blood vessels supplying the heart muscle by the age of thirty-five. This may result in an imbalance in blood supply to the heart; the supply of oxygen reduces while demands rise precipitously. This can have adverse medical consequences, such as heart attack (*myocardial infarction*) or sudden death resulting from abnormal heart rhythms. Using a small shovel, working slowly, and avoiding wet snow can reduce effort.

EXERCISE GUIDELINES

Exercises that involve moving the entire body over a distance are preferred for younger individuals at a reasonable level of fitness and health. These activities end with the suffix '-ing.' For example:

Walking
Jogging
Cycling
Swimming

These activities, often called *aerobic exercises*, are particularly efficient ways to burn energy and improve cardiovascular fitness. Playing, walking, and swimming in a pool will increase energy expenditure further because water provides much more resistance than air. However, swimming does not promote bone mineralization because it does not involve weight bearing.

A schedule can be made in order to exercise at the same times on a regular basis. The aim should be consistency. The individual can start or progress at any suitable pace. It will be easier to start gradually: exercise for short periods, such as fifteen minutes at a time, and progress to a half hour or forty-five minutes a day, three or four times a week. Continue the activity for as long as an hour if effort is very light. Reduce the time allotted to the activity as effort increases. Vigorous exercise can be limited to twenty minutes a day.

Weight-bearing exercises can be added to the regimen of older teenagers and young adults to increase both muscle strength and bone density. This will establish better bone mass by age thirty, after which there is an age-related loss for the rest of our lives. A formal weight-training program for strengthening bones is not necessary for children since many are already involved in activities such as jumping, climbing, and skipping. However, there is a well-documented age-related decline in physical activity during adolescence that will need to be addressed through a more systematic approach. A recent study found a sixty-to one-hundred-percent decline in energy expenditure through leisure-time physical activity in girls aged nine to eighteen years.

There is no universal exercise prescription or regimen for everybody. Be prepared to alter the program based on age, fitness level, the season of the year, and changing interests. Make the personal program productive. Goals can be accomplished around the house and at work that will incorporate increased physical activity. Good illustrations of this include the following examples: a teenage son or daughter using a reel mower to cut while father trims and edges the lawn.

Washing the car regularly by hand. Gardening or raking leaves in fall (especially appropriate for many seniors). Gardening on a regular basis is an excellent way to promote muscle strength and flexibility. It also involves weight bearing. An elderly individual who is already quite active may start light swimming or water treading in a swimming pool, generally remaining on the shallow side. Sedentary individuals can start with brief walks on level surfaces. Many of the health benefits of exercise in mature individuals appear with frequent, regular walks. Regular walks can be incorporated during lunch breaks at work. Elevators can be avoided to make more use of stairs.

Another factor that should be taken into account is the time of day during which physical activity occurs. We are all more vulnerable in the early-morning hours. This is believed to be due to the daily morning surge of a hormone called *adrenaline*, which is released from the adrenal gland. Adrenaline, which is also called *epinephrine*, affects the electrical activity of heart muscle, making it more susceptible to dangerous rhythms. The clotting cells of the body, called *platelets*, also are more apt to bond to form a *thrombus* upon arising. Blood pressure is also highest in the early morning. We believe that all these factors interact and account for the prominent clustering of heart attacks, strokes, and sudden deaths observed during the morning hours.

TELEVISION AND COMPUTERS

The subject of television viewing is commonly encountered, especially when dealing with families that have children. This medium can be a valuable source of information, news, and cultural activities. Unfortunately, it is seldom used as an educational tool. Instead, family members frequently choose animated cartoons, soap operas, movies, sitcoms, and game shows. Ironically, many "sports fans" invest hours watching football, basketball, and hockey, yet these same individuals rarely participate in any organized sporting events themselves. Television viewing is the number one "activity" following occupational duties for a large segment of society, having replaced sports and hobbies.

It also curbs interaction among family members and it is not uncommon to find multiple sets in a single household all in use. Children may have their own sets in their bedrooms. Not only does viewing replace other forms of activity, it has also been found to lower the level of spontaneous physical activity to rather unnatural levels. Thus we would use more energy just sitting not engaged in any particular activity.

This medium can be used wisely to our advantage by restricting the number of viewing hours and by making good choices in the programs watched. Unfortunately, discipline of this type is beyond the scope of most families as a unit. The result is a cycle of conflicting program choices, prolonged viewing times, tension, arguments and a collective loss of control. A radical solution to this problem adopted by some families is to eliminate television from the home altogether. This is an approach that works well in some cases. Another approach is to cancel cable or satellite connections in order to reduce the number of choices. In this way, rental movies and news items can still be watched.

The location of the set is also important. It is best not to have it in the family room or other rooms that are used heavily. Instead, it should be placed in a relatively isolated spot in the house where a special effort has to be made to engage in this activity. Consumption of meals and snacks while watching should be forbidden.

Parents who have made decisions of this type seldom regret the results. Their children now have more free time after school to learn new skills with their parents, and they will be more proactive in making friends who are already playing outdoors. Another advantage is that they have time for boredom now. Some degree of boredom fosters performance of independent tasks and creative thinking. Thus as parents, we may find that they spend extra time and effort on that science project, homework, or hobby.

Computers share some of the same pitfalls as television. Many youngsters use them purely as a source of entertainment and the educational potential remains unrealized. The responsibility to regulate children and ensure they use computers appropriately lies with the parents. Different parents will adopt different strategies, and there is no set formula that is guaranteed to succeed. Computer games should be selected so that they promote problem-solving to stimulate intellect. Repetitive tasks should be avoided. The total amount of time spent using computers on a daily basis should be controlled in young children, leaving time for social interactions and physical activity. At the same time, we will need to help develop computer skills and encourage research for factual information.

Families may find it increasingly difficult to regulate these types of activities at home, especially as children become adolescents. The school system can help by committing more time to structured physical activities. Unfortunately, there has been a decline in money, time, and effort devoted to sports activities in schools, which is partly responsible for the poorer health of children today.

DECONDITIONING

When exercise is discussed, many people will complain of fatigue. They complain that they are chronically tired—certainly, too tired to become involved in any formal exercise program. It is helpful to explore the basis of their fatigue.

Organic problems need to be ruled out, but for most of us chronic fatigue is just due to the plain stresses of everyday life. Just about everybody has these. The human body was not designed for the mechanistic ritual of modern life along with all of the positive and negative outcomes that this entails. It is still designed for 6000 BC. It reacts to sensory overload, prolonged concentration, or physical labor with primitive reflexes and emotions, such as fatigue. Unfortunately, the body's defense mechanism against fatigue remains equally primitive—stock up on calories. These are primitive reflexes, hard-wired somewhere deep in our limbic systems. It is important for us to understand this if we are going to work with our bodies rather than against them. That there is a natural tendency to turn to food following prolonged stress should be recognized. Alternative strategies can then be explored and planned. These will differ from individual to individual.

Having said that, for most of us, really the opposite is true. We are tired because we are chronically deconditioned. We will feel *more* energetic *if* we exercise. A healthy body weight will help make physical activity easier. Being deconditioned does not necessarily mean having excessive body weight. It can refer to poor exercise tolerance, poor muscle tone and strength, and a tendency to get shortness of breath soon after mild exertion. We can become deconditioned fairly rapidly following an illness or surgery as well.

A common basis for chronic fatigue that is often overlooked is sleep disorders. We will complain of sleep deprivation when we find ourselves missing the seven or eight hours per night to which we are accustomed. Modern-day occupational schedules frequently result in lost sleep during the workweek that tends to be recovered on weekends. This is the reason many of us sleep in on the weekends. However, this leaves us tired at the end of most weekdays. The physician will take this opportunity to review good sleep hygiene. The problem is considerably worse in shift workers, since it is really not possible to adapt to the alternating sleep schedules.

On the other hand, retirees and homemakers habitually retire to bed too early. These patients will complain that they suffer from fragmented sleep and frequently awaken at about four or five o'clock in the morning. They do not feel rested as a consequence. It is helpful to point out that these individuals are trying to spend too much time in bed. They will experience better quality of sleep if they limit their time in bed by retiring late and arising at an early, preset time.

Anxiety disorders are a common yet overlooked basis for chronic fatigue. This heterogeneous group of disorders affects more than ten percent of the population. Perhaps the most common of these is *generalized anxiety disorder*. The symptoms include excessive, uncontrollable anxiety or worry about a number of issues, irritability, sleep disturbance, difficulty concentrating, and fatigue. Lifestyle changes that can be invaluable for controlling this disorder include regular exercise and avoidance of caffeine and alcohol.

There is a tendency to consider fatigue as a physical condition that precludes exercise. As we have seen, for many, it is due to common mental and emotional states such as stress, sleep disturbances, anxiety, and depressed mood. Finally, there is ample medical evidence to show that regular exercise will improve all these conditions.

EARLY BENEFITS

There are several tangible benefits of regular exercise. In addition to weight control, it will improve the level of physical fitness and conditioning. This translates into better skeletal muscle tone and strength as well as a stronger skeleton. Studies have found that this promotes better mobility and fewer falls in the elderly, as well as fewer fractures when they do fall. A physically active lifestyle in children and adolescents significantly increases peak bone mass, which provides protection from osteoporosis later in life. The ability to regain bone with exercise after it has been lost due to age and sedentary lifestyle is limited.

Physical fitness helps improve cholesterol (more about this later) and blood pressure, protecting against atherosclerosis and reducing the incidence of heart attack and stroke. Regular exercise helps prevent the onset of diabetes even when body weight does not change. Many of these benefits of exercise can have an impact on general survival rate even when the obese individuals fail to lose weight. Deaths due to heart disease are reduced in smokers who are physically active even when they continue to smoke. A supervised exercise program has also been shown to reduce death rate following a heart attack.

For most of us, there are real benefits that begin on day one. Exercise promotes sleep and induces a feeling of well-being. Exercise on a *regular* basis translates into a sustained improvement in mood. As mentioned earlier, this means less anxiety and depression as well. The benefits of exercise in reducing stress are well known. This can have a significant impact on families and co-workers as well. Large corporations sometimes provide fitness centers in order to reduce tension and increase productivity in their employees.

Appreciate that the most difficult part of the exercise program is getting started. Conversely, the first item that gets eliminated from the routine, especially when there is disruption, is exercise. The decision to increase the level of activity remains the client's responsibility. They will need to schedule exercise into the daily routine. They should think long-term. There is no point in doing something for two weeks and then abandoning it. They will need to think of activities that they can enjoy today and many years from now. The regimen should not feel like work; it should be fun.

A useful approach in motivating teenagers to take up an active lifestyle is to exercise together as a family unit. Parents influence their children's behavior best by setting examples and routines. Competitive sports will also help hold their interest. Nowadays many couples have delayed child-bearing into their later years, typically when they are in their thirties. This will have a negative impact on their ability to enjoy an active lifestyle with their kids when they reach the pre-teen or teen years.

CASE HISTORY

RB, male
Age: 46 years.
BMI: 23

Looking back at the teen years, I did not practice any dietary restrictions. I used saturated fats such as butter freely and did not avoid fried foods. However, visits to local fast food outlets were not the norm, and most of the meals I consumed were home-cooked. I allotted considerable time to sports in high school. I also played on amateur soccer teams after school. I was not overweight at any point in time.

Sports and fitness were neglected during medical training and my work as a medical physiologist. This is unfortunate and it illustrates the problem of losing total control over one's lifestyle, which can be fostered by rigorous teaching programs and certain occupations. Leisure time was limited and largely spent recovering lost sleep and overcoming fatigue. This was certainly a very unhealthy lifestyle.

The dietary routine that I have followed for the past fifteen years limits consumption of fatty foods. This means avoidance of deep frying at home, omitting butter on bread, grilling or boiling fish and meat, and avoiding commercially-baked products such as pies cooked with lard. I have tried to increase fish consumption to one or two servings weekly. I avoid deep-fried battered fish.

My meals are comprised predominantly of grain products, vegetables, and limited servings of meat. I consume one or two glasses of skim milk daily or alternatively, yogurt and fat-free cheese. I will often eat fruit at the beginning of the meal. Most of my meals are not followed by dessert. If I do have one, it is a small helping only. I restrict very rich desserts such as ice cream to one or two small servings a month.

I avoid eating excessive amounts of salt by removing the saltshaker from the table, adapting to the natural taste of foods by salting lightly during cooking, and limiting commercially-prepared soups and pickles.

I have an active lifestyle involving dozens of household activities, such as mowing and washing cars. I feel that this is where I expend a large number of calories. I frequently shovel snow in winter, against my better judgment. This type of outdoor activity in cold weather increases energy expenditure further since the body has to use calories in order to maintain temperature. I am careful to increase consumption at meals in order to prevent weight loss.

My exercise routine consists of lifting weights and using a gym machine at home two times a week. I do not believe in converting the home into a fitness center or investing a lot of money into machines of this type. Instead, I have a low-end weight machine that cost no more than four hundred dollars as well as four pairs of dumbbells (total cost, two hundred dollars). I do not approve of a large monetary investment because, more often than not, these devices remain unused in basements. Instead, I focus on a schedule and a routine that I can live with. Personally, I do not like using barbells, since it requires holding a heavy weight up against gravity before any exercises are started. I find this stressful and unpleasant.

I exercise about an hour after awakening, before any breakfast is consumed. I am not sure that this is a good time for a middle-aged male to exercise from a cardiac point of view. My routine is to perform a few stretches followed by use of the gym machine. I start with low weights, using the high pulley for the upper body, bench press for the triceps, and the knee extension for the quadriceps muscle. I proceed to various arm exercises with the dumbbells. Since I have suffered a significant injury to the knee, I sit down when I perform arm exercises. I find that flexing the knee joint and avoiding complete extension is also helpful.

Following this, I perform exercises for the abdominal muscles. Initially, these were sit-ups, which I found quite unpleasant. I have replaced these with the "bicycle maneuver," where one lies flat on the back and peddles the legs in the air. This is an excellent alternative to sit-ups. After a full sequence of these, I return to the gym machine and repeat the stations using heavier weights.

I limit my routine to twenty or twenty-five minutes, two times a week. Any more would be more like hard work and unsustainable. I now avoid competitive sports due to age-related factors and the condition of my knee. I find that a home weight-lifting routine permits good control over the muscle groups that one wants to exercise while minimizing injury.

A routine of this type has led to increased upper-body musculature and controlled any tendency to gain fat in the middle. My BMI has increased slightly but still remains in the healthy range. I do not suffer from high blood pressure. I am a non-smoker, and alcohol consumption is limited to three or four ounces weekly.

COMMENT

This case history shows that medical information can be incorporated into daily lifestyle decisions in order to prevent weight gain and related health problems.

6

Practical Strategies for Weight Control

FOOD LABELS

The ability to read food labels is a useful skill to develop. The widespread availability of nutritional information on food labels is a useful means to regulate weight. The three main sources of energy in our diets are carbohydrates, fats, and proteins. The energy obtained from each gram of these substrates is as follows:

Carbohydrates	4.0 Calories
Protein	4.0 Calories
Fat	9.0 Calories

The average North American gets fifteen percent of the daily energy requirements from protein, thirty-four percent from fat, and fifty percent from carbohydrates. In some localities in North America, almost fifty percent of daily energy is derived from fat! In some parts of the world, the quantity derived from carbohydrates exceeds that from protein and fat.

Nobody really knows the ideal mixture, but everybody agrees that there are drawbacks at extremes. A high fat diet has been implicated in accelerating atherosclerosis and triggering premature heart disease, strokes, and cancer. Excessive protein intake aggravates kidney problems. However, a high carbohydrate diet is sometimes linked to protein deficiency, lack of adequate minerals and vitamins, and diabetes. In turn, diabetes is a powerful risk factor for premature death and disability.

For many of us in North America, protein deficiency is not an issue (the one large exception is the very frail elderly population). The minimum daily protein requirement to meet losses is forty grams. Health-care workers recommend somewhat more in order to avoid deficiencies in essential amino acids. Compare this with the figure for actual protein consumption in an individual consuming 2,200 Calories: eighty grams. An individual suffering from severe class-3 obesity, consuming 6,000 Calories daily, will consume 230 g of protein per day!

The recommended amount of calories derived from fat for most individuals is twenty to thirty percent of the day's total energy intake. One can remember this number at the grocery store and try to ensure that each individual food item falls within this guideline. This will prove to be an extremely useful tool in our armamentarium. However, also take the total amount of fat into account. For example, a specific item may have only twenty percent fat content, but the daily requirements of fat may still be exceeded through ingestion of large quantities of the same item. Conversely, some items can be high in percentage fat but have very low total fat content and contribute negligible amounts to the daily intake.

Let me illustrate these concepts with the example of a glass of water. It lacks fat and calories. If we placed a drop of vegetable oil in the same glass, the percentage of the total calories derived from fat in this item increases to one hundred percent. In spite of this, the contribution that this glass of water is going to make to the day's energy intake is still close to zero. It is generally recommended that adult women consume a maximum of sixty-five grams of fat per day, and men eighty-five grams.

Unfortunately, milk fat levels listed on labels are not as clear as they should be. They are expressed as a percentage of the total volume, which results in low numbers. This is misleading, since milk is almost ninety percent water. These values should be expressed as in other foods, that is, as a percentage of total calories obtainable from that product. We would find that regular milk, which is labeled 3.25% fat, yields *almost fifty percent* of its calories from fat.

Carbohydrates are a relatively small source of energy on a weight basis. A continual source is vital to provide energy for the nervous and muscular systems. Restriction of sugars and starches forces the body to convert fat and protein into *glucose*. This also results in the formation of acidic substances called *ketone bodies*. Daily energy intake from carbohydrates can be increased to fifty-five to sixty percent from current values, with a corresponding reduction in fat, in individuals at a healthy body weight.

Carbohydrate-rich foods often have indigestible components that do not provide energy but help provide a sensation of fullness and control constipation. They are often associated with water. For example, an apple is almost eighty-five percent water. In contrast, fats do not dissolve in water and tend to be more concentrated. Many food items that are rich in protein also have significant amounts of fats.

LACK OF RESULTS

Exercise will also stimulate appetite; therefore, a combination of exercise and judicious eating habits is essential in maintaining or losing body weight. Some individuals will spend an hour at the gym, swimming, or jogging in the evening and then go to the nearest fast food outlet for a hamburger because now they are hungry and they feel they deserve a treat. Let us review some numbers. On average, we burn five hundred Calories by jogging for a whole hour, which is not an easy task for anyone. Unfortunately, one commercial hamburger alone that is ingested in less than five minutes will yield five hundred Calories, effectively neutralizing one hour's hard work. This is the reason clients will complain that they lead physically active lifestyles and yet do not lose a pound. They are certainly telling the truth, but they need to pay attention to their appetite and food choices. It also illustrates the futility of trying to exercise off an unhealthy diet.

THE HUNGER INSTINCT

I often ask patients whether they feel hungry when they are preparing to retire for the evening. The answer is often in the negative. Daily cycles of hunger and fullness are rather natural events for the human body, although not always pleasant ones. It is not inappropriate for these autonomic reflexes to re-establish themselves. In fact, slimmer individuals experience them on a daily basis.

There is an abundance of food in modern-day society, and eating times have become totally habitual. Hunger as a cue for meal times is frequently downplayed as we regulate our lives around social and occupational obligations. However, food intake should be reduced until there is a recurrence of hunger. Carbohydrate and fat stores will be mobilized during these episodes.

A useful observation is that the sensation of hunger does not intrude appreciably into the sleeping state. This is analogous to the situation where a physician advises a patient to take certain troublesome medications before retiring in order to avoid unpleasant side effects, such as nausea. Hunger at the end of the day, when all the day's calories have been ingested, signals that more energy has been expended than consumed and the body is ready for more. One effective behavioral cue is to perform nightly oral hygiene (brushing and flossing) earlier, say right after supper, at six o'clock, signaling that one will not snack into the evening. The same sensation is relatively blunted at breakfast time as well.

A variation on this strategy would be to go hungry by consuming lighter meals during busy periods of the workday, when attention is directed to other matters. Alternatively, one could exercise during these periods. It is surprising how the sensation dissipates during physical exertion. Again, none of the latter strategies works as well as going to bed hungry because all the day's meals have already been consumed. Typically, if one comes home from the office at suppertime famished and tired, it would take an enormous amount of willpower to eat a light meal. An individual might be able to do this two or three times, but not consistently over a long time. Very unpleasant strategies are unsustainable.

This does not imply that meals should be omitted. This would be a very undesirable state, placing a burden on the body. Invariably, it results in loss of control and overeating at the next meal. A habitual pattern of this type can only aggravate weight gain. The hormonal stresses that result from this type of dietary pattern are explained in chapter seven. Research findings show that individuals who habitually consume breakfast are less likely to become obese or diabetic.

DIETARY FAT

Dietary fat is the most highly concentrated form of energy in food. It is also the way our body stores excess calories and is the main tissue deposited around muscles, internal organs and under the skin in obesity. It is important to limit excessive consumption of fat in the diet. This is good advice for many individuals. It is relevant to weight-reduction or attempt to maintain weight by slimmer individuals and those who have suffered a heart attack or stroke.

Another benefit is that lower fat intake also reduces the risk of cancer. Researchers have attributed twenty percent of cancers to obesity. Some of the increased risk may be due to increased consumption of fat. Slimmer individuals may have a relatively higher consumption of fruit and vegetables, which may account for some of the differences in risk of cancer.

Let us explore specific examples and strategies. Try to increase the variety of food consumed on a daily basis, at the same time substituting lower-fat choices for richer recipes. This is now easier than ever with the widespread availability of cookbooks specifically dealing with lower-fat recipes. Also, the availability of diverse foods in supermarkets has improved enormously over the last two or three decades. Consider the availability of tropical fruits and vegetables in stores as well as ethnic cuisine in supermarkets and restaurants. Select products labeled low fat, low in saturated fat, calorie-reduced, or light, if you choose not to calculate fat and energy content. This is less desirable, since some of these products may have less fat but not fewer calories. Similarly, products may be labeled "light" when they have reduced fat content compared to the regular version but they may still be very fatty. Common examples include salad dressings used for sandwiches, peanut butter and ice cream.

When preparing meals, limit added fat and explore substitutes. Select vegetable oil such as olive (technically a fruit), sunflower, or canola oil, and soft nonhydrogenated margarine when fats are required. Limit frying, which converts potentially beneficial forms of fat, such as vegetable oil, into harmful ones. Unfortunately, many families continue to rely on this method of cooking on a daily basis. It has been cited as a common problem in immigrants from less affluent countries, where sophisticated cooking techniques and equipment are not available. In any case, a simple strategy is to make greater use of ovens, non-stick frying pans, and grills, where the fat is continuously drained away. Adopt low-fat cooking techniques including broiling, baking, microwaving, and steaming. Do not add fat when cooking meat, since it releases its own during the cooking process. Use a paper towel to blot away any fat visible on meat after cooking is complete.

I would caution readers not to extrapolate these rules to children unless there is an obvious problem and a physician has had a chance to examine the child. Again, the expertise of a dietitian may be required. Children require adequate amounts of fat in their diets for the growth spurt as well as a dense energy source for a high level of physical activity. Excessive limitation of fat in the diet can result in deficiency of *essential fatty acids*, which the body cannot synthesize, as well as loss of fat-soluble vitamins such as vitamins A, K, D, and E.

VERY FATTY FOODS

Commit items that have highly concentrated amounts of fat to memory and try to limit them. Important examples are listed.

Butter, margarine, or mayonnaise

Oil

Cheddar cheese

Chicken, breaded and fried, with skin

Chocolate

Bacon

Croissants, Danishes, donuts, or muffins

French fries

Potato chips

Peanuts, roasted in oil

Peanut butter

Pie or cake

Sausage

A single serving of these items can add an additional ten to twenty grams of fat. Approximately sixty to seventy percent of the calories obtained from peanut butter are derived from fat. Regular cheese contains sixty to ninety percent fat calories. Likewise, a hot dog wiener has seventy percent fat calories.

SATURATED FATS

Limit excessive consumption of saturated fat. Research early on showed that this type of fat was particularly harmful when dealing with lipid profiles and blood-cholesterol levels. Similarly, harmful fats, sometimes referred to as *trans-fatty acids*, are also derived from vegetable oils via hydrogenation. These are commonly found in commercially-prepared convenience foods such as French fries, cookies, deep fried foods, and crackers. Younger individuals usually have a high consumption of these types of fats. This occurs at a time when many youngsters do not have a clear appreciation of, or commitment to, these issues. In these cases, parental guidance is appropriate.

Many people still have the misconception that the most important substance to avoid in their diets is cholesterol. In other words, they believe that a lower cholesterol intake will lower their blood-cholesterol levels. A relationship between blood-cholesterol levels and cholesterol intake does start to appear at higher values, but again, the relationship is clearer for saturated fats. The consumption of three or four eggs a week is still compatible with a cholesterol-lowering meal plan. Each egg contains about 200 milligrams of cholesterol. Eggs that are rich in omega-3 fatty acids are now widely available. Cholesterol is not found in foods of plant origin.

The term saturation refers to the chemical changes in fat substances that make them more linear and they align in a more regular fashion. Therefore, saturated fats are solid at room temperature. In contrast, unsaturated or polyunsaturated fats are non-linear. This is useful information in and around the kitchen, allowing one to look at the fat and deciding whether or not it is saturated.

Vegetable cooking oils are liquid at room temperature and are polyunsaturated (good) fats. However, compare this with the fat found on red meat; it is more solid (bad). Here is another rule of thumb: saturated fats are derived mainly from animal sources. There are some notable exceptions that are worth remembering. For example, oils derived from tropical plant sources, such as coconut and palm, have been found to be high in saturated fats. Another useful observation is that the unique fats found in fish sources have "heart healthy" properties. They have been found to reduce coronary events but, of course, remain an important source of calories in the diet when weight control is an issue.

Physicians are interested in the bigger picture. They want to address all the health and lifestyle concerns a patient may have and will avoid making broad inflexible statements regarding nutrition. Personal preferences are always taken into account. This is an evolving field, and useful and healthy properties are being discovered in many foods that were previously discouraged. Some researchers have proposed that milk has cancer-preventing properties. For example, studies have linked higher milk consumption with a reduced risk of breast cancer. Egg yolks have several important micronutrients. Eggs are an excellent source of protein at the extremes of age, young and elderly. However, eggs are not recommended in infants younger than one year of age due to their allergic properties. Recent research consistently shows that the consumption of nuts—including peanuts, which is actually a legume—is beneficial. On the other hand, fruit, which is frequently recommended for cancer prevention, can be contaminated with pesticides, potentially posing a health hazard. Similarly, one cannot reasonably ascribe extraordinary preventative or therapeutic properties to any one food item or supplement. Nutrition is just not that straightforward.

Let us return to some strategies that can help lower saturated fat and cholesterol consumption. Many of the foods listed in the table above are culprit. Limit high-fat foods such as deli meats, sausages, high-fat cheese, butter, lard, and cream. Other foods include organ meats (liver, kidneys, sweetbreads, brain), shrimp, crab, lobster, egg yolks, poultry skin, hydrogenated margarine, tropical oils, and hydrogenated fats found in potato chips, crackers, and cookies. The serving size of meat and poultry should be limited to the size of a deck of cards. Lean cuts of meat should be chosen and all the visible fat trimmed away. Salads can also be fatty when rich dressings are used. A Caesar salad has much more fat than a carefully prepared meat sandwich.

SALT CONSUMPTION

An additional advantage of regulating food consumption and maintaining an appropriate body weight is that salt intake can be reduced. Many recipes include not only generous portions of fat but also salt. Salt (sodium chloride) is a major component of body fluids. Sodium is the main ion in extracellular fluids, which includes blood. Without it, most food would be too bland to enjoy. Excessive amounts are commonly found in commercially-prepared foods, fast foods, pickles, and sauces. The daily recommendation for sodium is less than 3,000 mg for the general population. Lower values are recommended for individuals with high blood pressure. In more practical terms, one teaspoon of salt is six grams of sodium chloride and 2,400 mg of sodium. However, the actual intake is considerably higher in many individuals, especially males.

A chronically high intake of salt leads to water retention in the body. This increases filling in the circulatory system, sometimes resulting in elevated blood pressure. In some individuals there is leakage of fluid into the tissues in dependent parts of the body, such as the feet. This is called *peripheral edema*. In this way, excessive intake is linked to high blood pressure, or *hypertension*, which is a potent risk factor for heart and kidney disease.

Overweight individuals may be able to normalize blood pressure by reducing salt intake and losing weight. In many cases, hypertension is not caused by excessive salt ingestion, but can be aggravated by it. Often, physicians can control hypertension using fewer medications when their patients lose weight.

Spices or lemon juice can be substituted to add flavor to food. Read labels and try to select unsalted fresh, frozen or canned vegetables, and unsalted nuts. Gradually reduce the use of salt while preparing meals in order to develop a taste for natural flavors.

DAIRY PRODUCTS

Use dairy products carefully. Dairy products are a good source of calcium, animal protein, magnesium, zinc, potassium, vitamin B12, phosphorous, riboflavin, and essential fatty acids. Milk, but not yogurt and cheese, has added vitamin D. A glass of milk has 300 mg of calcium and 100 IU of vitamin D. The average daily intake of calcium in the United States is 600–800 mg. Milk is an important source of water, promoting good hydration. Dairy products are well-suited for growing children, providing them with an easily-absorbed source of calcium and energy derived from fat.

Family physicians face significant challenges with the consumption of dairy foods. It is widely acknowledged that intake of dairy products is often inadequate in the years critical to bone mineralization. We often find that milk consumption declines during the growth spurt for girls (ages eleven to fifteen) and boys (twelve to eighteen). Consumption of soft drinks increases. In addition to being a calcium-deficient substitution for milk, soft drinks contain phosphates that can bind calcium and further inhibit calcium uptake in the intestine.

Sometimes we see overweight children who show significant differences in eating habits. One group of adolescents may exhibit "overnutrition." This means that they consume excessive amounts of all food groups. They will report generous intakes of cheese and ice cream along with four or more glasses of milk on a daily basis. Dietary histories in others reveal obesity secondary to excessive consumption of energy-rich, nutrient-poor products. Interestingly, this latter group of individuals may have lower levels of intake for minerals and vitamins such as iron, calcium, zinc, folic acid, and vitamins C and D.

It is quite common to see inappropriate parental concern when dealing with children's eating habits. Parents will bring their twelve-year-old son into the doctor's office, alarmed that their child is gaining excessive weight. After an appropriate history and physical examination, the physician may reassure them that this is a normal maturational stage for their son. Generally, boys gain weight just before their growth spurt. At this time, their lower bodies (feet and legs) have elongated but their trunks are still foreshortened, accentuating the uptake of fat tissue. In the years following this "fat spurt," the upper body grows rapidly while fat stores disappear and muscle appears.

A common complaint regarding many girls is that they are fastidious eaters and too lean. Again, reassurance from the physician may be all that is needed along with an explanation of normal female maturation. It is helpful to point out that these children do not demonstrate any lack of energy in play and sports. Girls tend to deposit fat stores during puberty. It is important to stress that concerned parents not override the body's signals for hunger and satiety. This may result in poor eating habits and obesity later in life.

An interesting problem involving milk is also encountered in infants. A child may come to a doctor's notice at one and a half to two years of age when mother complains that the infant is a poor eater. The history may reveal that the infant is consuming excessive amounts of cow's milk, often refusing to give up the bottle. One typically encounters an infant who appears well-nourished but pale. Often, the blood count reveals iron deficiency anemia. This phenomenon has been termed the *milk-baby syndrome*. It appears to result from baby's reluctance to adapt to table food, which requires significant hand-eye coordination and some effort. The infant prefers instead to run around with a bottle in hand.

CALCIUM AND VITAMIN D

The reader can see that the physician cannot adopt a one-size-fits-all approach. He or she will need to take a detailed dietary history and individualize the approach. Extra care will be required when dealing with the consumption of dairy products in children. Dairy products are the best sources of calcium and vitamin D. Recommendations for these will vary according to age, sex, lifestyle, and family history.

An important feature to take into consideration when prescribing vitamin D supplementation is geographic location, since this vitamin can be produced in the skin with the help of sunshine. For example, I often recommend supplements of vitamin D to seniors during the months of October to March in Canada, when both dietary sources and ultraviolet light are inadequate. In more southern areas, fifteen minutes of sunlight exposure on bare skin stimulates enough vitamin D production for the whole day. Other risk factors for a low vitamin D status include a vegan diet, remaining indoors for prolonged periods, excessive use of sunblocks, and having darker skin. Dietary sources of this vitamin include milk, margarine, fish oil, and egg yolk.

Vitamin D increases the absorption of calcium from ingested food as well as from the kidney. It also helps to promote bone mineralization. Adequate amounts of calcium and vitamin D help reduce the rate of bone loss that is observed after age thirty-five.

There are several risk factors for osteoporosis in addition to calcium deficiency and inadequate vitamin D status. These are aging, female sex, small body build, low body weight, heredity, Caucasian or Oriental race, sedentary lifestyle, alcohol consumption, cigarette smoking, and early menopause.

Returning to the issue of weight control and the consumption of dairy products, we can expect good results from our efforts, since this food is a major component of the daily diet. A notable exception is among Orientals, where there is a higher prevalence of *lactose intolerance* and for whom milk products are not an important part of the daily diet. Milk and yogurt with one percent fat or less are good choices. Another is fat-free sour cream. Limit two-percent milk, fat-reduced cheese, and frozen yogurt. Avoid whole milk, cream, ice cream, and regular cheese. It is important to note that skim milk is low in fat but not calcium. Again, I would not impose any of these restrictions to adolescents unless confronted with overnutrition and obesity. If one cultivates the habit of choosing leaner dairy products, then a significant impact can be made in the long-term in a relatively comfortable fashion.

The picture becomes more complicated upon further examination. One may find that when limiting fat from dairy products, we will turn to other sources for satiety. These sources may consist of hydrogenated fats found in pre-prepared snacks, products that are often calcium-deficient. It would be more appropriate to substitute other nutritious food products, such as fruit, grain, and cereal. Another worrisome finding is that diets high in calcium and dairy fat may be linked to prostate cancer. In a recent eighteen-year study, milk and calcium intake during menopause were not associated with a reduced rate of hip fractures. Instead, adequate levels of milk consumption during childhood and adolescence, and vitamin D intake during menopause lowered the risk of osteoporotic fractures. In women, dairy products have been linked to a reduction of breast cancer. Finally, adequate calcium intake has been linked to blood pressure improvements as well.

A list of vegetarian sources of calcium was provided in chapter two. You should be aware that recommendations for the consumption of dairy products in adults is a controversial topic in academic circles. The physician can work with the client after their personal choices have been made.

Passive Strategies

Control availability. We all need to regulate easy access to rich meals, since there is a natural biological drive to eat. This is a sad state of affairs at a time when large populations of the world do not have adequate nutrition.

Let us deal with some parental concerns first. It is not uncommon to come across parents who complain that their two-year-old is a fussy eater. Sometimes the dietary inquiry will reveal that the infant drinks unnecessary amounts of juice, which inhibits appetite and fulfills caloric requirements. The physician points this out and advises restriction. Some parents will have already tried this, unsuccessfully. A much better way to accomplish the goal is to stop keeping bottles or cans of juice in the house. The child quickly learns to adapt to the available food choices. Similar advice is often given to families with older children when parents complain of excessive consumption of junk food. You are going to have a fight on your hands if the kitchen cupboards are stacked with salty fried snacks or desserts. Expecting kids to resist tempting foods is asking too much.

The same principles can be useful to adults. They can make it a point to avoid keeping fatty snack foods in the kitchen. Once these products make it into the home, it is unreasonable to expect people to resist time and time again. Keep fruit, yogurt, and cereal handy for these occasions. Adopting this type of passive approach should work on a long-term basis to regulate the age-related gain in body weight, helping to keep the middle-age spread at bay. The partner's help can often be enlisted if he or she does the grocery shopping, making this an even less uncomfortable experience. Partners should participate on a life-long basis in weight control, promoting healthy eating for the whole family.

Affluent clients and personnel with certain job constraints pose a significant challenge. These individuals will point out that their occupations require that they be away from their homes for more than twenty-four hours at a time, forcing them to eat in restaurants. Affluent individuals also go out to dinner with colleagues and clients frequently. Professional gourmets prepare exquisite meals that are served in very pleasant atmosphere. Availability of rich meals is unrestricted, while constraint becomes difficult. The body's signals of hunger and satiety are overridden. The more one is involved in this subculture, the greater is the difficulty maintaining a healthy lifestyle. Few make use of the hotel swimming pool or spend the evening in the fitness center. This lifestyle is going to require a firm commitment to one's goals.

We have to think back to the basics: the energy balance equation. For all of the evenings spent in this manner, there is going to have to be a more rigid fitness program. This will provide longer time commitments burning calories. One should try to make better food choices at these get-togethers, avoiding really fatty servings, deep-fried dishes, and rich desserts. Smaller portions can be chosen. If there is a weight problem, it may be a lot easier to avoid these events altogether. Alternatives can be suggested to colleagues that do not involve commercially-prepared meals or excessive alcohol consumption. Finally, these events can be restricted so that they are few and far between and have essentially zero impact over the long term.

There are a few things one can do following occasions of this type. Invariably, appetite will be curbed for one or two meals immediately following one of these events. Heed the body's signals and take advantage of this. Make the next meal exceptionally light, accompanied by a large drink such as water, fruit juice, or skim milk.

RESTAURANT DINNERS

On a similar note, limit restaurant meals. It is very difficult to control food choices in this environment. Assume that commercially-prepared meals will have abundant portions of fat and salt to keep customers coming back for more. Most consumers are not going to eat salads while everybody else is enjoying tastier meals.

There are several ways to address this. One approach is to study the menu carefully to try to come up with the best choices. There may even be heart-healthy dishes listed separately. Some facilities may provide the fat content of their selections on the menu. Failing this, another approach is to customize the meal. For example, one may request that the mayonnaise and butter be omitted from sandwiches, or may choose to avoid deep-fried side dishes, creams, and gravy. The number of egg yolks should be reduced in breakfast dishes. Similarly, it is entirely acceptable to eliminate the butter from toast and bagels and apply jam or fat-reduced cheese directly. Continental breakfasts are particularly problematic if the wrong choices are made. The size of the portions of both food and calorie-rich drinks can be limited by making individual requests.

Eating habitually in restaurants will require considerable discipline in order not to disrupt one's program of personal fitness. It can be done, but again, a more passive approach will be easier. This lifestyle should be avoided if possible. Alternatively, one could bag meals. Even if one meal was prepared at home and carried to work on a daily basis, unhealthy choices would be reduced significantly. A final option is to increase energy expenditure by more vigorous exercise, such as lifting weights on a regular basis. This is practical for younger adults only.

SUGAR CONSUMPTION

Another significant source of energy intake is the simple sugars found in many commercially-prepared foods. Some researchers have suggested that obesity is increasing in North America at a time when fat intake is declining. Excessive intake of simple sugars is now believed to be a major source of calories. Even though simple sugars are relatively low in energy compared to other foods, large amounts become significant and aggravate weight gain.

Many individuals habitually consume carbonated soft drinks on a daily basis, and it is not unusual to encounter patients who report intakes of a liter (about three cans) or more. A twelve-ounce (360 ml) can of soft drink contains ten teaspoons (forty grams) of sugar, which provides 160 Calories. A youngster who drinks four cans a day gets more than twenty-five per cent of the entire day's energy requirements from sugar! Water, which is entirely devoid of energy, is no longer a popular drink in today's society. The consumption of soft drinks now exceeds milk consumption in most adolescents.

Drinks such as milk shakes can also add hundreds of calories to the meal due to their fat and sugar content. Alternative strategies include providing unsweetened or artificially-sweetened drinks. Sugar substitutes can also be used in yogurt and jams. Certainly, the consumption of beverages is encouraged to maintain hydration. It is also a useful approach to consume a large low-calorie drink with the meal to help achieve a sensation of fullness earlier. Good hydration with sugar-free beverages is also linked with better dental health. The elimination of water as a beverage deprives us of the dental benefits of fluoridated water.

Commercially-prepared foods again emerge as a major culprit in the excessive consumption of refined sugar. The largest consumers of these products are children and adolescents. Ingredients such as sucrose, maltose, dextrose, fructose, maple syrup, corn syrup, honey, and corn sweetener all refer to related products. Sugar found naturally in fruit is called *fructose*, and milk sugar is called *lactose*. A common problem is the inclusion of excessive amounts of refined sugar in everyday prepackaged food items. Simply put, a single serving of given product may contain five teaspoons of sugar when many consumers would be satisfied with only two. The option to add more could be made available to the consumer for many products. I suspect that once a taste for higher amounts of sugar has been acquired, it tends to become the reference level for other items.

The medical literature lists refined carbohydrates as another unhealthy component of our Western diets. Having said that, there is still no medical consensus on the full impact of these carbohydrates on well-being. Some individuals associate refined sugars with a host of daily ills, including lethargy, hyperactivity, irritability, yeast infections, menopausal symptoms, and so on, but the evidence is lacking. There is evidence linking it to *Crohn's disease*, an inflammatory disease of the bowel. This does not necessarily mean that avoiding sugar can prevent Crohn's disease.

Refined sugar lacks fiber, minerals, and vitamins but contains a ready source of energy. Brown sugar is a good source of iron. Extra energy in this form ultimately converts into fat for storage. The consumption of calories in this form occurs at the expense of complex carbohydrates found in grains, which are rich in indigestible fiber and micronutrients. It is important to limit carbohydrates as well as fat in order to achieve weight loss. Many products that are fat-reduced have almost the same number of total calories as the regular version due to the addition of simple sugars. These sugars will convert to fat in our bodies and there will be no net benefit.

Extra care is required when selecting cereals, ice cream, soft drinks, and baked products for youngsters. It is totally unacceptable to allow them to make their own uninformed choices at the grocery store. I often advise new mothers to limit sugary products for their infants. Heath-care providers look forward to the time when the food industry exercises responsibility when including sugar into food, as they already have for fats. Perhaps what is really lacking is a strong drive from the medical profession.

Healthier fats

All fats are not the same. Fats come from a variety of sources and have been found to have differences in terms of their effect on our bodies. However, the total number of calories is the same. Each tablespoon (fifteen milliliters) of fat contains 120 Calories and contributes fourteen grams regardless of the type of fat. It is not difficult to choose oils and fats that are low in saturated fat.

Monounsaturated and polyunsaturated fats appear to be healthier. Olive oil is a particularly good choice, since it contains more than seventy percent monounsaturated fats. In contrast, butter is more than sixty percent saturated fat, while coconut is almost ninety percent. Almonds have less than ten percent saturated fat, containing mainly polyunsaturated and monounsaturated fats. Almond and walnut consumption have been associated with fewer heart attacks and deaths in recent studies. These are best consumed raw or dry-roasted, not fried. Fats derived from fish sources called *omega-3 fats* have also been linked to increased life expectancy. Products such as olive and canola oil are good sources of essential fatty acids as well. Hydrogenation reduces the content of essential fatty acids from these food sources.

Fats improve the taste and enjoyment of food and are important physiologically because they signal and maintain a sense of fullness after a meal. These particular fat choices can be used to our benefit to supplement the meal. However, relatively small quantities should be chosen from this food group when weight maintenance is an issue.

DESSERTS

Limit desserts. Recognize that the consumption of desserts is a custom or habit. Most of us acquire this habit in childhood, since it is commonplace to offer sweet items as a reward to children. In this way, positive associations with the consumption of desserts develop over time. However, this can be changed fairly easily.

Avoiding dessert will help limit the number of unnecessary calories consumed at the meal as well as the amount of fat and simple sugars. A large helping of dessert can add one half to two thirds of the total energy consumed at a meal. Small quantities of sweet dishes are acceptable on occasion. Unfortunately, many people tend to snack on rich desserts on a regular basis. An easy way to limit these calories is to avoid having this food item in the home. It requires time and effort to prepare these dishes yourself.

Meals can be organized so that the leaner and healthier fare is consumed first. For example, the meal could start with a generous helping of fruit. Richer dishes could be eaten later and desserts omitted altogether. The portions of these food items should be reduced if necessary. In this way, the bulk of the meal is formed by fruit, vegetables, and grain products in satisfying portions.

7

Weight Control and Diabetes

THE METABOLIC SYNDROME

Physicians have recently recognized a group of symptoms and signs that occur in overweight and obese individuals. Common problems include fluid retention in the extremities, high blood pressure, abnormal lipid values, and abnormalities in the regulation of the blood sugar, glucose. We believe that the habitual consumption of excessive calories results in high levels of insulin in these individuals. Some individuals have a genetic predisposition to these conditions as well.

Insulin is a hormone released by the pancreas, a gland located just behind the stomach and the first part of the small bowel. Insulin promotes storage of glucose, deposition of fat, and retention of salt and water in the kidneys. High insulin levels in the body eventually lead to desensitization of insulin receptors and a resistance to the metabolic action of this hormone. These changes have been termed the *insulin resistance syndrome* or the *metabolic syndrome*.

The individual who suffers from this disorder is typically approaching middle age, very overweight, and complains of fluid retention in the ankles. Physicians will identify the other abnormalities through an examination and blood work. The physician may discover hypertension, high blood sugar, increased triglycerides, and low HDL cholesterol. Typically, the patient has abdominal obesity. This disorder predisposes patients to diabetes and premature heart disease, and the diagnosis is well worth pursuing.

Studies suggest that one in four Americans already suffers from the metabolic syndrome. The prevalence of diabetes is about twelve percent. Furthermore, up to fifty percent of diabetics in the United States may be unaware of their condition.

These statistics parallel our findings with hypertension, where more than twenty-five percent of the adult population suffers from the condition but fully one-third of those are not aware of it. These figures are worse when lower cutoff values are used to define high blood pressure, as recent publications have proposed. Elevated blood pressure damages vital organs and eventually leads to heart attacks, heart failure, kidney failure, strokes, and blindness. Since high blood pressure is not associated with any symptoms, it has been called "the silent killer." Finally, tobacco must be avoided completely, since it interacts with all these underlying conditions and worsens the prognosis.

DIABETES

The final outcome of these changes is called *diabetes mellitus*. The term mellitus is mentioned sometimes in order to distinguish it from a totally different disorder, called *diabetes insipidus*. There are two types of diabetes involving blood sugar, or glucose, regulation. These have been called type I and type II.

In *type I diabetes*, there is an injury to the pancreatic gland resulting in a critical decline in insulin secretion. In turn, this leads to *hyperglycemia*, which is the medical term for high, uncontrolled levels of glucose in the blood. Insulin is the main hormone signaling glucose availability, helping tissue utilization and storage. Since glucose requires water to dissolve, it also draws fluids from tissues, all of which are lost from the kidneys. Thus we have a situation where the body is starving for its key energy supply while calories are being voided in the urine. Fat stores are mobilized to produce an alternate source of energy, called ketones. Common symptoms of this disorder are weight loss in spite of increased hunger, unexplained weight loss, thirst, frequent voiding, slow healing of cuts, and yeast or fungal infections. Other symptoms include fatigue and blurred vision.

The loss of fluids in diabetes results in deficits of important stores of potassium and magnesium along with significant dehydration. Potassium and magnesium are two of the most abundant ions found within cells. They are involved in nerve and muscle function. In addition, magnesium is vital for the proper functioning of hundreds of chemical reactions in the body. Depletion of potassium and magnesium results in weakness and abnormal heart function. Magnesium depletion can cause muscle spasms. Magnesium can be replenished by dietary sources including whole grains, legumes, nuts and seeds, chocolate, green vegetables, some seafood, poultry, avocados, bananas and some berries. Good sources of potassium are peas, spinach, carrots, potatoes, tomatoes, and mushrooms, as well as fruits such as bananas, kiwis, oranges, avocados, raisins, melon, prunes, and pumpkin. However, potassium losses can be life-threatening and hospitalization is frequently necessary for correction. Other medical conditions are associated with high blood-potassium status and the physician will recommend avoiding these items in the diet. Potassium levels in the blood must be measured to help the physician decide the appropriate approach to the patient.

Type I diabetes occurs secondary to the production of antibodies directed against the pancreas. Antibodies may be triggered by viral infection. Often, there is a genetic predisposition. It has a tendency to develop early in life, usually childhood to early adulthood. The symptoms and signs develop relatively quickly. After several decades, the patient may develop disease in the small blood vessels, leading to loss of vision, kidney disease, and threatened limbs.

In contrast, *type II diabetes* is related to obesity in many cases. More than ninety percent of diabetics are in the type II category. As we noted before, there is chronic stimulation of insulin in these individuals. The problems associated with this were discussed above. Finally, there is desensitization in the body to the insulin so that one finds the same loss of glucose control seen in type I diabetics. Calories are wasted in the urine. This is associated with lipid abnormalities and premature heart disease. Life expectancy is shortened by a decade.

Diabetes is associated with two types of complications, called *microvascular* and *macrovascular*. Microvascular refers to a disease of the small blood vessels that eventually leads to kidney disease, impaired vision, and peripheral nerve damage. In this way, diabetes is the leading cause of kidney failure and blindness in affluent countries. *Macrovascular* disease refers to progressive atherosclerosis in the bigger blood vessels, which eventually leads to coronary artery disease, strokes, and impaired circulation in the legs. Diabetic patients are more likely to suffer early mortality from premature heart disease than from microvascular complications. Research has shown that the control of blood pressure and abnormal lipid profiles helps reduce death from heart disease, whereas tight control of blood sugars delays progression to microvascular complications.

Type II diabetes is diagnosed through blood tests. The exact recommendations for screening vary, but some risk factors include being over forty-five years old, obesity, having a first-degree relative with diabetes, being a member of a high-risk ethnic group, the presence of hypertension and heart disease, and diabetes during pregnancy.

These serious metabolic problems are now starting to appear in children. Medical research has discovered abnormalities such as high-fasting insulin levels and reduced sensitivity to insulin in overweight children. Children are also exhibiting high blood pressure related to obesity. These findings reinforce our concern for this health epidemic, and we must all take weight problems in childhood seriously. The initial approach will be to control diet and increase physical activity.

We are not in a position to prevent the onset of type I diabetes, but type II disease is often related to lifestyle. This is true not only in terms of onset but also progression to life-threatening complications. Even to this day, the cornerstone of treatment of type II diabetes remains diet and exercise. Less than ten percent reduction in body weight is associated with lower blood pressure and improved blood-sugar control. A diet that is low in fat and simple sugars helps control blood sugars, while exercise helps large organ systems such as muscle utilize the glucose. In effect, these organs act like sinks. The diet is developed on an individual basis through meetings with a dietitian, while the medical doctor develops a comprehensive treatment plan. Generally, insulin is provided in the form of injections to patients who have type I diabetes. The medical treatment of type II diabetics is usually started with a class of medications known as *oral hypoglycemic agents*.

A dietary program will emphasize the need to lose excessive weight and maintain a healthy body weight. This can even normalize blood sugars. Small, frequent meals are recommended in order to help insulin handle calories. Limit the amount of simple sugars found in foods such as white rice, white bread, potatoes and pasta. Better alternatives include whole-grain products and oats. However, a common finding is that patients place exclusive emphasis on sugar and starch consumption. Fat intake should also be addressed.

In keeping with many of the same guidelines for healthy eating, adequate amounts of fiber, vegetables, and fruit should be consumed. Include the peel of the vegetable if possible. Also, make more use of lentils and legumes. Fruit has high amounts of natural sugar, which should be limited. Thus, smaller helpings should be consumed. Fruit juice has most of the pulp or fiber removed, which will promote rapid uptake of the sugars in the digestive system. Small quantities of juice are acceptable. Alcohol consumption will make it more difficult to regulate blood sugars. Artificial sweeteners can be used in beverages and baking. Reduce the meat or protein portion of the meal to about one quarter of the plate. Experiment with meatless recipes and choose leaner cuts of meat. Skin should be removed from poultry. Meat can be broiled, barbecued, microwaved, steamed, or roasted—avoid frying if possible.

Exercise and an active lifestyle are crucial for adequate control of blood sugars. However, as with diet, exercise will have to be planned carefully. This is a concern in patients who are being treated with insulin or oral medications for diabetes. Bursts of unplanned activity can lower sugars rapidly, resulting in depletion of the brain's main nutrient and loss of consciousness. This is called a *hypoglycemic reaction*. This is a medically urgent situation that can be treated with oral intake of juice, regular (not diet) soft drinks, or tablets containing simple sugars before glucose levels become too low. The signs and symptoms of *hypoglycemia* include pallor, mood changes, confusion, tremor, sweating, dizziness, blurred vision, headaches, fatigue, and hunger. Sugars should be checked before and after vigorous effort for these reasons. Type I diabetics can reduce their insulin or consume extra calories before working out. Hypoglycemia is a major limiting factor in our ability to regulate blood glucose to target levels. If blood sugars are too high, exercise is not advisable until medical treatment corrects the problem.

There are important medical concerns in our diabetic population when addressing lifestyle issues. We know that the risk of cardiac disease increases significantly in diabetics. Often, the symptoms of heart disease are masked or atypical, delaying the diagnosis. This is partly related to abnormal functioning of the autonomic nervous system, commonly found after one has had diabetes for several years. This can be a dangerous combination that can lead to very serious complications, including death, in individuals who undertake an exercise program without proper consultation. Physicians will arrange exercise stress testing in asymptomatic patients frequently. Similarly, the family doctor should be notified if any unusual symptoms develop.

Many patients with heart disease are on an important and useful class of medications called beta-blockers. Examples include metoprolol, propranolol, atenolol, acebutalol, and nadolol. These drugs block the body's response to increased adrenaline or epinephrine levels, thus sparing the heart from dangerous levels of stimulation. However, the hypoglycemic reaction involves the release of the same hormones. In this way, the body's reactions to low blood sugars, including hunger, palpitations, and tremors, are impaired. We call this *hypoglycemic unawareness*. Patients may not recognize the warning signals of low blood sugar and may lose consciousness before they can help themselves. Extra care will be required with the use of these medications.

Another important concern that involves younger patients is the deliberate wasting of calories in order to lose weight. We find that some teenagers may reduce the dosage of insulin, which triggers some of the metabolic derangements seen in uncontrolled diabetes. This is a very serious problem that should be discussed openly with the health-care team. The patient is taking serious health risks, including loss of potassium and water, and acidifying body fluids. All the long-term consequences of diabetes are also accelerated.

CASE HISTORY

CM, female
Age: 50
BMI: 38, now 28

I was diagnosed with diabetes in February of 2000. This did not really surprise me since my mother also suffered from it. As with my mother, I was very overweight and already had a diagnosis of high blood pressure. I knew that the first thing that I had to do was change my diet. I stopped eating sweet foods such as chocolate bars, pies, and cookies. I knew that this was not going to be easy, but it had to be done. I then spoke to my family doctor, who gave me a food guide to get me started until I could meet a nutritionist. I started to lose weight almost instantly, but not too fast, by following the guide. Two weeks later, the nutritionist provided a 1,500 Calorie diet for me. She inquired about my activity level, likes, and dislikes and the manner in which I prepared my meals. I told her that I had stopped frying as well. I knew that I was on the right track.

I had not been an active person before the diagnosis. I did not want to go on diabetic medications and had to do something about my activity level. In March, I got a job cleaning our bank. This added another hour of light work to my work at home. I started to walk outdoors as well when the weather improved in the spring. The walks increased when my daughter came home from university in April. It was not always easy, since I was so heavy, but the more weight I lost, the easier it became to walk. I lost fifty pounds by September and needless to say, I was quite pleased with myself.

When I get hungry between meals, I eat a piece of fruit or raw vegetables. I treat myself on weekends to snacks that I really enjoy, such as potato chips. I do not want to deprive myself of these treats. I had lost seventy pounds by December.

I also stopped smoking in April 2002. Everyone knows that this increases weight. I try to eat low-calorie foods or chew sugarless gum when I get the urge to smoke. I bite into an apple rather than a cookie when I get an urge to eat. I also find that walking helps to control appetite and the craving for nicotine, both of which I do not feel will ever go away completely.

I think that I have done well. I ate everything that I wanted to for fifty years. It is still not easy, and I do not tell myself it ever will be. You do what you have to; no one can do this for you. And I try to keep busy.

COMMENT

As a physician, I am quite proud of CM, who has demonstrated that progression of type II diabetes can be controlled through lifestyle changes. In addition, she addressed her addiction to tobacco successfully.

Unfortunately, the treatment of type II diabetics is frustrating for physicians and patients. Most patients fail to normalize their body weight for complex reasons. Dietary guidelines may be a part of the problem. Historically, physicians placed the emphasis upon avoidance of simple carbohydrates. The emphasis shifted to the so-called prudent diet with fewer calories, more complex carbohydrates and reduced fat. Recently, researchers have demonstrated greater reductions in body weight and better blood sugar control with a very low carbohydrate (25%), high protein (45%), and high fat (30%) diet. We do not know the full impact of these types of diets on the progression of diabetes, kidney disease, heart disease or life expectancy.

Compliance with dietary guidelines outside the framework of research studies is a significant problem. I have been able to discontinue the use of insulin in obese type II diabetics using a diet that is low in simple carbohydrates, fat, and total calories in hospitalized patients. This is followed by a complete loss of control over body weight and a return to insulin administration shortly after the patient leaves the hospital setting. The emphasis has shifted to treatment with medications since there is a large body of evidence supporting their efficacy.

8

Alcohol and Tobacco

ALCOHOL

Alcohol consumption is an exceedingly complex phenomenon in today's society. There are benefits as well as drawbacks to the use of this agent. This is not an issue that family physicians can ignore, since this drug is used so commonly in North America, if not the entire world. It is estimated that more than ninety percent of adult Americans have used alcohol. This highly addictive drug is here to stay and actually forms an integral part of our culture. It is ubiquitous in social and business gatherings and is often consumed by individuals in their private time.

BRAIN CHEMISTRY

Alcohol, or *ethanol*, is classified as a *depressant*, which means that it suppresses the centers of the brain that determine alertness and sensory awareness. In addition, it is known to have a disinhibitory effect, interfering with executive centers that regulate higher cognitive function and emotion. This property is highly valued by people since it reduces acute anxiety, induces a state of relaxation, promotes socialization, and enhances pleasure. Of course, at higher levels of intake, sedation becomes overwhelming, resulting in sleepiness.

It is a common pattern to use *caffeine*, which is a *stimulant*, in the early hours of the day to promote wakefulness, eliminate fatigue, and enhance cognitive function and even athletic performance. Common sources of caffeine include coffee (140 mg per cup), tea (50 mg per cup), colas (40 mg per 12 oz), and chocolate bars (40 mg per bar). Caffeine has a synergistic action with stimulatory hormones in the body. The most important of these chemical mediators is *adrenaline* (or *epinephrine*), which is released by the autonomic nervous system as well as the adrenal gland. Adrenaline levels increase with stress as well. This hormone increases alertness, heart rate, and skeletal muscle power. People consciously or unconsciously use caffeine to promote all these functions in order to achieve their goals during the day.

Alcohol users exhibit a behavioral change during the latter part of the day, whereby activities take advantage of the sedative properties of ethanol. These behaviors include drinking wine with the evening meal, having a drink or two at the local bar following work, or having a nightcap. The physiology of each of these activities is exactly the same; we are now suppressing the stress reaction that we had been promoting earlier. Euphoria is believed to result from rapid changes in levels of alertness, which is regulated by the brainstem. In this way, the cyclic use of caffeine and alcohol provides some degree of euphoria in a controllable form that is legally sanctioned and socially acceptable. In other words, we are manipulating brain chemistry.

Arguably, these behaviors may help us cope with the unnatural lifestyles and stresses imposed by modern living. It may enhance our lives by promoting pleasure, albeit short-lived. Medical researchers have found recently that moderate alcohol consumption is associated with increased life expectancy, possibly by improving HDL cholesterol and reducing clotting, thereby lowering the rate of heart disease and heart attacks. This relationship is seen when alcohol consumption is two or three ounces per day in men and one or two ounces in women. This relationship does not hold true at lower or higher levels of consumption, and it does not apply to younger adults. Formerly we believed that this property was unique to wine, which has *flavonoids*. Similar compounds are found in red grape juice and tea. However, recent evidence supports a protective effect for other forms of alcohol as well.

THE BURDEN TO SOCIETY

While our understanding of the impact of alcohol upon lifestyle is anecdotal, there is no dearth of information illustrating the damage that this drug causes to the human body, families, and society. After all, this is a highly addictive drug. The markers of *addiction* include: loss of control, compulsive use, craving, and adverse consequences, that is, use despite harm to the individual. An analysis of the cost of addiction to this agent to society is beyond the scope of this review. However, let us return to the issue of weight control and the direct impact that heavy alcohol consumption has upon the human body.

Ethanol is metabolized in the body and generates energy or calories. As discussed before, excess calories are converted and deposited in the form of fat in adipose tissue. This aggravates abdominal, or visceral, obesity. Similarly, there is deposition of fat around the heart, liver, and other internal organs. Transportation of fatty acid molecules derived in this manner results in *hypertriglyceridemia*, which is a risk factor for heart disease.

The risk of bleeding in brain tissue, a condition called *hemorrhagic stroke*, is increased. In addition, alcohol is directly toxic to most organ systems in the human body. It is known to damage peripheral nerves, brain cells, heart cells, liver cells, and so on. Some medical terms that describe the result of organ damage of this type include *alcoholic dementia, hepatitis, cirrhosis, pancreatitis*, and *cardiomyopathy*. Alcohol interferes with the normal pacemaker of the heart, resulting in abnormal rhythms, typically after a weekend binge. This phenomenon is called *holiday heart syndrome*. Alcohol has a direct inhibitory action on heart muscle, which can precipitate *congestive heart failure* in individuals who already have structural damage from heart disease. Chronic consumption of alcohol also results in hypertension. Many individuals can normalize blood pressure by abstinence, making medications unnecessary in these situations.

Alcohol is classified as a *teratogen*, which means that it can adversely affect the developing fetus when the mother drinks during pregnancy. There is an established link between alcohol consumption and breast cancer in women. Drinking affects sleep quality, which can interfere with alertness during the day. In this way, it can affect drivers indirectly along with the direct effect on coordination and judgment. As mentioned earlier, it relaxes the muscles about the throat area, increasing snoring and lowering blood-oxygen levels. This property can aggravate the imbiber's susceptibility to heart disease. It is associated with aggressive cancers of the head and neck as well. The reader can appreciate that these are extremely serious disorders with a high degree of morbidity and mortality.

Acutely, consumption damages the lining of the stomach and breaks down the protective barrier to acid, resulting in a condition called *gastritis*. Consumption of excessive amounts of caffeine, acetylsalicylic acid-like agents, and smoking aggravate this problem. This can lead to bleeding in the upper digestive tract, which can be life-threatening. It is especially disconcerting to see teenagers drinking alcohol, since it is more detrimental to the developing nervous system.

Heavy alcohol users may exhibit unusual nutrient and mineral deficiencies. For example, clinicians will discover deficits in magnesium, thiamine, folic acid, and other B vitamins. Magnesium deficiency is uncommon in healthy individuals since it is found in many different foods (good sources were listed in chapter seven). Thiamine is vitamin B1. It plays a vital role in the ability of the body to use carbohydrates for energy. The body does not store this vitamin well, so it is important that sources are included in the daily diet. The best sources of thiamine are pork, liver, peanuts, milk, and fortified cereals. Folic acid deficiency interferes with the production of blood cells. Deficiency of the B group of vitamins damages nerves in the arms and legs, a condition called *peripheral neuropathy*. These patients will complain of abnormal sensations in their extremities or difficulty walking.

Some drinkers use alcohol to alleviate symptoms of anxiety disorders and depression. They appear to experience a brief respite from their symptoms immediately following drinking. However, this property is temporary since alcohol has well-known adverse effects on mental health.

ALCOHOL AND ENERGY

Each gram of ethanol generates seven Calories, which exceeds the energy obtainable from sugar. The amount of energy in a drink of wine (7 oz), spirits (1.5 oz, made with 6 oz soft drink), or beer (12 oz) averages 150 Calories. Four drinks will provide the same number of calories found in a complete meal.

Low amounts of alcohol stimulate appetite, promoting some degree of loss of control over hunger and excessive consumption of food. Poor food choices may be made in this state. Appetite is curbed at higher amounts of alcohol intake. There is a corresponding reduction in intake of most minerals and vitamins as well. Changes in the cells lining the digestive tract interfere with their ability to absorb nutrients. Chronic ingestion of these "empty calories" eventually results in obesity and aggravates nerve and tissue damage as described above. Even though advertisements associate drinking with youth, socialization, and popularity, continued intake eventually results in a body habitus that resembles older individuals with osteoporosis, excess fat, and weak muscle tone. This is hardly a desirable image for our youth.

What is the position of the family doctor, given all the complexities of this drug? Physicians cannot promote alcohol consumption when dealing with teetotalers because it is heart-healthy. Alcohol is a highly addictive agent that can be damaging to the patient, the family, and society, resulting in more harm overall. Family doctors will inquire and document responsible intake without passing further judgment.

The medical profession adopts a more proactive position when confronted with alcoholism. The patient is provided with appropriate medical information and referrals are made to a team of dedicated nurses and physicians specializing in addiction. There is no medical "cure" for alcoholism, and success is contingent upon patient motivation and participation. It is especially distressing to encounter individuals who use the drug heavily without regard for their health. Sometimes physicians will refer to this behavior as *chronic suicide*.

The problem that I have with the concept of moderate consumption of this agent is that the daily intake of two to three drinks is going to impair one's ability to think clearly, operate a motor vehicle, interact with loved ones, or be productive in one's free time. Personally, I think this is too high a price to pay. This is a decision that each one of us has to make for ourselves. It is conceivable that new agents may be discovered that will share many properties with alcohol but lack the adverse effects on the nervous system and other organ systems.

Tobacco

What are some of the everyday concerns of smoking in general, and with respect to weight control, in particular? Tobacco smoking invites a powerful addiction to the chemical *nicotine*. Like alcohol, this is a legally-sanctioned drug. Ironically, it is also the most lethal drug in common use the world over. Fortunately it is becoming less and less socially acceptable. Unlike alcohol, cocaine, or opiates, it does not cloud consciousness, induce euphoria, or trigger hallucinations. It is not linked to motor vehicle accidents or domestic violence.

Disorders related to tobacco

Nicotine is a potent stimulator of the autonomic nervous system, which controls the body's basic functions at an unconscious, or involuntary, level. These activities include blood flow and digestion. The overall result is to decrease blood flow to the digestive organs and extremities.

Nicotine interferes with the metabolic machinery residing within the walls of blood vessels, a layer called the *endothelium*. Thus, it causes *endothelial dysfunction* throughout the body. In this way, tobacco use is linked with premature atherosclerosis, heart disease, stroke, *abdominal aneurysms*, and *peripheral arterial disease*. More lives are lost due to cardiovascular disease related to smoking than from tobacco-related cancer. Tobacco smoke is responsible for over ninety percent of the cases of *chronic obstructive pulmonary disease* due to its ability to increase mucous production in the airways and obliterate lung tissue. It is linked to cancers at various sites including lip, mouth, larynx, esophagus, lung, bladder, pancreas and kidneys. The greatest avoidable risk factor for heart disease and cancer remains cigarette smoking. Smoking represents a risk to both mother and fetus during pregnancy and is linked to fetal death, premature delivery, smaller babies, and developmental delay. It is associated with osteoporosis. Smoking along with sunlight exposure are the two leading causes of premature aging of the face. Smoking cigarettes is also associated with poor dental health.

NICOTINE AND BODY WEIGHT

Nicotine is classified as a *stimulant* because of its effects on the central nervous system. Therefore, it can aggravate anxiety disorders. As such, it also seems to be linked to a lower incidence of depression. Attempts to stop the use of this drug may precipitate depression during the withdrawal reaction. Unfortunately, this accounts for the continued urge to use this drug in some individuals.

Another property shared by psychostimulants of this type is reduction of appetite. Smokers tend to be thinner, and there is a real tendency to gain weight after quitting. However, smoking should account for only a ten-pound weight difference in these situations. Some individuals gain considerably more body weight with time after successfully stopping the use of tobacco. It is believed that they are resorting to food for oral gratification. Mood disturbances are linked to derangements in appetite as well. Most patients report an increase in appetite after stopping tobacco use. I usually advise patients to try and stop smoking before asking them to address any weight concerns.

There are several medical options when attempting to quit smoking. I will not review them here. However, bupropion is a novel approach that may be of special interest to those predisposed to depression. It is marketed as an antidepressant as well.

Physicians cannot condone the use of tobacco under any circumstances given the medical evidence. Likewise, individuals should not continue using this drug in order to suppress appetite.

CASE HISTORY

HL, male
Age: 39 years
BMI: initially 38, now 30

Two years ago, I arose at eleven o'clock in the morning to prepare for my shift at a construction site. I was scheduled to work from four o'clock in the afternoon to eleven o'clock that evening. I started to experience a burning sensation in my chest and upper back as I was getting ready. It would last only a few minutes at a time and I put it off as heartburn. By the time I arrived at the worksite, the burning feeling turned into a burning pressure. I felt it in my chest, lower jaw, and down both arms. I started to develop shortness of breath and I broke into a cold sweat. I knew that I was in trouble. My co-worker called 911 and I was taken to a hospital.

The doctors said that I had suffered a heart attack caused by a blocked artery. I was sent to a larger hospital for angioplasty.

I realized that it was time to wake up after having had a heart attack at age thirty-seven. I was smoking a packet of cigarettes a day and was overweight. I had a lot of bad eating habits and weighed 235 lb. I usually drank fifteen to twenty bottles of beer on the weekends. It was time to change my lifestyle. I read a lot of material and realized that many foods that we eat work against us. My family doctor and I came up with a plan to change my poor eating habits. I started to eat and drink differently during the three-month recovery period. Nowadays, I eat three meals daily, which I feel is very important. My wife and I make sure that they are nutritious. I stopped drinking pop and other drinks that are high in sugar. The meat that we buy is always lean. All these changes help keep the weight down. There are times when I cheat, but not often, because I know what can happen.

I had done shift work for fifteen years, working days one week followed by nights the next. I believe that shift work played a big role in the heart attack. The body never gets a chance to adjust working like this and doesn't recover. This realization led me to change jobs.

I have been staying active for two years now. I have changed jobs and altered the way I was eating. I feel like a twenty-year-old again. My weight is steady, at around 190 lb. We can eat most of the things we like in moderation. I can function and have a lot of energy with a healthy low-fat diet. I have reduced my smoking to eight or nine cigarettes a day and I no longer drink alcohol. I am fully recovered and enjoy life to the fullest. I am also taking medications for heart, blood pressure, and cholesterol.

COMMENT

HL has premature heart disease. There was a strong family history of elevated cholesterol and his lifestyle did not help matters. He is correct in pointing out that work habits can contribute to heart disease. Medical research has shown that shift workers suffer from heart disease earlier and have increased mortality. Our patient waited for six hours before seeking help. He had dismissed the symptoms as heartburn. This is a common error that is potentially very dangerous. The definitive treatments for heart attack are more effective the earlier they are administered; in other words, "time is muscle." I would like to see further weight reduction and cessation of smoking. He also had an unhealthy pattern of drinking, binging over the weekend.

This case describes a late presentation of heart disease. Typically, young males have little interaction with health-care professionals until serious problems of this nature arise. There is a corresponding reduction in opportunities to identify and investigate health-related concerns or discuss preventative medicine. Men also exhibit more risk-taking behavior. These are important public health issues that have not been addressed successfully. Women visit physicians more often due to various requirements, including contraception, screening for sexually-transmitted diseases, screening for cervical cancer, pregnancy, childcare, mood disorders, and autoimmune conditions.

9

Medical Implications of Lifestyle Changes

INITIAL SCREENING

Consult a physician before starting an exercise program. You will find this recommendation everywhere. However, it is somewhat problematic. The family doctor may order an electrocardiogram following a physical examination, but a normal interpretation does not mean that the heart is normal. Family doctors cannot rule out significant blockages in blood vessels supplying heart muscle, a condition called *coronary artery stenosis*, in office visits. This would require fairly sophisticated testing and a referral to a specialist.

We can obtain a more accurate medical clearance using an exercise stress test, which will show us how the heart is functioning under a workload. It will reveal whether or not there are areas of heart muscle that are getting enough oxygen when the subject is running on a treadmill. If there is a suspicious result, further, more invasive testing may be recommended. However, cardiac events can be unpredictable. An unstable atherosclerotic plaque can develop a fissure and develop a *thrombus*, or clot, leading to a heart attack. It would be too expensive for the health-care system to perform these types of assessments for every overweight or slim man or woman who wanted reassurance. Remember, also, that the risk to the individual increases from year to year.

What happens instead is that the health-care professional makes some general recommendations based mainly on knowledge and experience. Sudden death from cardiac causes is the initial presentation in about twenty percent of all heart patients. In other words, neither the physician nor the patient was aware that anything was wrong until this catastrophic event. A formal evaluation may be considered for individuals who are more than thirty-five years old with one or more risk factors for heart disease.

Tailor the exercise program to age, build, and fitness level. For example, if the client is an obese middle-aged male, he should not start playing basketball with thirty-year-olds. Heavy physical exertion has been shown to increase the immediate risk of heart attack or sudden death. The risk declines in physically active individuals. The physician can provide an exercise prescription that will include the target heart rate. Even if individuals demanded and paid for exercise stress tests, they still would not know anything about other aspects of health. Adverse medical outcomes due to exercise have become a public health issue. These mishaps have been dubbed the "Stone Syndrome" by the popular media following reports of a complication suffered by the film star. Finally, we still have to use some judgment. This applies to children as well. They can harbor physical ailments that go undetected until physical stress is added to the picture.

A thorough assessment is performed routinely on individuals who have suffered a heart attack. The medical guidelines here are clear. The exercise stress test allows us to divide patients into low, intermediate, and high-risk groups and to provide exercise prescriptions. The patient will need to be referred to a cardiac rehabilitation center for a supervised exercise program if he or she falls into the intermediate, or higher-risk, group.

HEART DISEASE

Familiarize yourself with the symptoms of heart problems. Excess body weight creates more work for the heart and promotes blockages. Physical exertion will increase the demand on the heart, resulting in a faster rate of pumping as well as an increase in the strength of contractions in order to send more blood and oxygen to exercising muscle.

Oxygen demand increases for heart muscle as well. When there is significant narrowing of the blood vessels supplying the heart, insufficient oxygenated blood reaches heart muscle. There is build-up of lactic acid, which stimulates local pain receptors. This pain is called *angina pectoris*. The quality of this pain can vary from person to person. It can be dull pressure, crushing, tightness, burning, squeezing, or heaviness. The severity ranges from mild to severe. It should not be dismissed because it is very mild and not bothering the patient that much.

The location is variable, ranging from the upper abdomen or stomach area to the lower jaw, shoulders, and the arms, down to the hands. The discomfort is deep—in other words, you cannot reproduce it by pushing on a particular spot on the chest or shoulder. It is called *visceral chest pain* for these reasons. It tends to be intermittent, lasting for a few minutes at a time. It is typically, but not always, brought on by exertion. Rest often relieves the discomfort. Generally, it does not have a sharp, jabbing, or cramping quality.

There may be associated symptoms, such as shortness of breath, faintness or dizziness, or profuse sweating. Swelling of the feet and shortness of breath when lying down are other clues. If any of these symptoms develop at rest or upon starting an exercise program, further exertion should be stopped and a physician consulted. Unfortunately, a lack of adequate oxygen to the heart can also be silent, that is, lacking any warning symptoms. This is commonly found in diabetics.

Many people believe that heart disease is diagnosed when the symptoms that have been described above occur. It is important for the public to appreciate that this disease has a long silent phase. Many of us start to deposit fatty material within the inner lining of blood vessels in early adulthood. This occurs for twenty or more years, until narrowing becomes critical and symptoms start to appear. Physicians normally expect to see symptomatic heart disease after age forty. It tends to occur approximately a decade earlier in men than women.

The risk factors for atherosclerotic heart disease include male sex, increasing age, positive family history of premature cardiovascular disease, smoking, diabetes, obesity, high blood pressure, high cholesterol, and a sedentary lifestyle. We all know of cases where patients deviated from this pattern and developed heart problems unexpectedly. Notice that the first three items listed are beyond our control; these are called the *unmodifiable risk factors*. However, the remaining are all *modifiable risk factors*. Recent estimates show that approximately eighty percent of adults have at least one modifiable risk factor for premature cardiovascular disease. Almost sixty percent of adults are sedentary.

MONITORING THE PULSE

Learn to monitor the pulse. This is probably the easiest personal method to determine level of physical fitness. Heart rate and pulse will be slower in physically-fit individuals. The physiological basis for this is that heart muscle becomes stronger and larger (hypertrophies) with fitness. It can pump more blood into the great arteries with less effort and fewer beats per minute. This applies at rest as well as during exertion.

The normal resting pulse rate is sixty to one hundred beats per minute (bpm). One often finds that physically-fit individuals have resting heart rates at the lower end of this range, for example fifty-five to sixty-five beats per minute. Sedentary, overweight adults will register rates of eighty to one hundred beats.

The easiest method to determine pulse rate is to press on the radial artery near the wrist. Run two fingers of the dominant hand along the thumb of the other hand on the palmar side. Slide the tips of the fingers to the level of the wrist and feel for a pulse. The pulse will be more prominent in slimmer individuals, where there is less interference by fat tissue.

Practice counting the number of beats for a full minute. Next, try to determine the pulse rate by counting for only ten seconds and multiplying by six to get the rate. This is important, because the heart rate will decline quickly after exercising when one stops to determine the pulse. The specific pulse rate for healthy individuals that will provide maximum benefit from exercise is listed according to age and fitness level below.

Age	Low fitness (bpm)	Higher fitness (bpm)
15–29	140	160
30–49	130	140
50 or older	120	130

The client will need to increase exercise intensity gradually in order to achieve the appropriate training rate to improve cardiovascular fitness.

Again, the rise in pulse with exertion will be diminished in very fit individuals. On the other hand, individuals who are very unfit may show large increases in pulse rate, reaching close to the maximum values listed above, by performing warm-ups! Coincident with this, there is also a rise in blood pressure, whereas pressure remains almost the same in fitter individuals.

Many heart and blood-pressure medications can modify the pulse or the rate of heartbeat. Two of the more important classes of these medications include *beta-blockers*, such as metoprolol, atenolol, and propranolol, and *calcium channel blockers*, such as verapamil and diltiazem. These medications protect the heart by reducing both the rate and the strength of contractions of the heart. In this way, the oxygen demand of the heart is lowered and the heart is protected. This is an extremely useful property of these agents in most cases. However, you cannot use your pulse response to assess exercise requirements or fitness. Heart attack patients will be given individualized instructions for pulse counts following their exercise stress tests. Initially, these will be much lower than the heart rate they reached during the stress test. Higher rates are to be achieved only under supervision.

LIPIDS

Learn how to interpret cholesterol levels. Many individuals find it difficult to appreciate the meaning of these numbers when the physician discusses them. Medical researchers continue to encourage the lowering of cholesterol levels through nutrition and physical activity as well as medications. This has translated into improved survival by reduction of heart disease and stroke. Physicians who have been in practice less than fifteen years have already witnessed these improvements. However, it is also true that overweight people can have low cholesterol levels and slim individuals markedly elevated ones. Genetics is also believed to play a role.

The complete fat, or rather, lipid profile consists of four values: total cholesterol; *high-density lipoprotein*, or HDL; *low-density lipoprotein*, or LDL; and *triglycerides*. The triglyceride component usually corresponds to fat stores in the body and can be elevated with obesity, diabetes, and alcohol consumption. The value should be less than two mm/L. Triglycerides have a smaller role in heart disease and stroke.

HDL cholesterol represents the cholesterol that is being transported from the blood vessels into the liver for excretion. It is often called "good cholesterol" because it is believed to reduce atherosclerosis. Epidemiological studies show improved survival at higher levels of HDL cholesterol. Unfortunately, males tend to have low HDL levels. Female hormones tend to raise the level, which appears to be responsible for the lower incidence of heart disease in women during their reproductive years. HDL levels should be greater than one mm/L. Exercise is a powerful way to increase HDL.

LDL cholesterol is commonly called "bad cholesterol" because it represents lipid that is being transported from the liver to the walls of blood vessels, promoting blockages. This value should be less than four in most individuals. However, in those already at higher risk for heart disease, it should be less than three. This can be achieved through weight control, exercise, good nutrition, and medications. An easy way to remember these numbers is shown below.

> HDL should be greater than 1mm/L
> Triglycerides should be less than 2 mm/L
> LDL should be less than 3 mm/L in high-risk groups
> LDL should be less than 4 mm/L in lower risk groups
> The ratio of total cholesterol to HDL should be less than 5

The numbers above follow the sequence one through five when the metric system is used. If you are more comfortable with the Imperial system, then multiply mm/L by forty to obtain cholesterol values in mg%. In this case, the recommended numbers change to: HDL greater than 40 mg% and LDL, less than 120 mg% in high-risk individuals.

Cholesterol levels do not correlate well with intake of cholesterol. Instead, saturated fats are a bigger culprit. These fats are used directly in synthesis of cholesterol. However, it is recommended that the daily intake of cholesterol not exceed 300 milligrams.

Here is a summary of the effects of different types of fats on cardiovascular risk:

>Omega-3 fat from fish: reduces clotting and lowers risk
Monounsaturated fats found in olive oil: lower LDL
Polyunsaturated fats found in vegetable oils: lower LDL
Saturated fats found in lard, butter, and coconut oil: increase LDL
Hydrogenated oils in vegetable shortening and hard margarine: increase LDL and cholesterol

THE MEDITERRANEAN DIET

I do not feel that it is realistic to advocate major alterations in dietary habits for everyone. However, some information that has been presented can be understood using the Mediterranean diet as a model. This is a term applied to the traditional dietary habits of people from Greece and Italy. Research in the early seventies established that this dietary pattern was associated with significantly lower rates of heart disease and increased life expectancy. Similarly, increased life expectancy has been linked to the traditional Japanese diet, which features soy products and fish.

The traditional Mediterranean diet provides about thirty-eight percent of its total calories from fat. The crucial difference is that there is a much lower consumption of saturated fats from animal sources than in the "Western diet." Instead, the diet is richer in omega-3 fatty acids, and monounsaturated and polyunsaturated fats. The diet consists primarily of fish, grains, vegetables, fruit, nuts, and olive oil. Red meat is eaten sparingly. It is useful for us to be aware of these types of dietary patterns and to try to adopt some of their features. In this way, unhealthy food choices will start to play a progressively smaller role in our daily dietary choices.

As a physician, I deal with the management of weight problems, hypertension, lipid and glucose abnormalities, and heart disease with medications on a daily basis. However, I am always fascinated when I learn that, in many cases, results from lifestyle changes match or exceed those obtained using our best medical treatment!

OSTEOARTHRITIS

You should appreciate the adverse medical consequences of exercise as well as the benefits. We are all continually given information regarding the health benefits of exercise, but there are negative factors that we should also bear in mind. We read about the exploits of well-paid professional athletes in the newspapers on a daily basis. However, the story of sports injuries suffered by amateurs and professionals alike largely remains untold. These injuries have a significant impact on the quality of life of these individuals. They can result in chronic pain and disability. In this way, exercise contributes to the significant prevalence of pain in society. It is estimated that twenty-five percent of individuals over the age of forty live with chronic pain, and this figure increases with age. Ironically, these injuries may preclude further participation in aerobic sports and promote a sedentary lifestyle.

Let me relate the experiences of one patient in order to illustrate this issue. This middle-aged male decided to enroll in a squash group in order improve his level of aerobic fitness and to control weight. He diligently learned the game by playing with the local squash club members and was soon playing on a regular basis. About a year later, he sustained a severe injury to the right knee while playing with a particularly aggressive player ten years his junior. The injury occurred when the opponent placed the ball into one of the rear corners of the court.

When attempting to retrieve the ball, the patient's forefoot hit the wall, twisting it laterally, or sideways, with great force. This resulted in severe pain, requiring the player to be assisted off the court. The knee immediately swelled to twice its normal size. There was gross instability, with the lower leg literally sliding ahead of the upper when the patient walked. The patient elected not to have surgical intervention to repair the damage and instead waited for nature to take its course.

The diagnosis in this case was a rupture of the *anterior cruciate ligament*, which is one of the main ligaments stabilizing the knee joint. In addition, there was pain in the medial or inside joint compartment, likely from a tear in the *medial meniscus*, which is one of the cartilaginous cushions of the knee. Needless to say, his squash career was over. Moreover, there was a significant *reduction* in his quality of life, since he lived in chronic pain. Similarly, he could no longer participate in games that involved jumping or running. Our athlete could not bring himself to take medications continually in order to remain pain-free. In this way, he joined the ranks of middle-aged individuals who live restricted lives due to self-imposed medical conditions. He discovered for himself that the knee is the most vulnerable joint in the human body. It turns out that the patient described above is the author.

Studies have shown that girls who play soccer are particularly vulnerable to knee injuries of this type and more likely to develop osteoarthritis in the injured joint as a result. Physicians are continually treating injuries associated with sports. These range from forearm and wrist fractures from falls sustained in skiing or rollerblading to head trauma and concussions suffered in baseball and eye injuries in racquet games.

Injuries of these types invariably sideline our sports enthusiasts. What is particularly devastating is that healing is often incomplete and these individuals suffer the consequences for several years, if not decades. I feel that it is important for physicians to discuss these issues in order to raise awareness of the pitfalls of exercising. Zealous statements emphasizing only the advantages of exercise are clearly not adequate. Individuals can make better choices about the sports activity they decide to embark upon and take the necessary precautions appropriate for that activity. Protective equipment such as helmets is an obvious case in point, but protection can only take you so far. Many other risks remain unchecked due to the nature of the activity. We often recommend swimming, which is easier on joints since there is much less weight bearing. Again, basic precautions are necessary. For example, drowning accounts for the second most common form of accidental death in children. Ironically, a person who knows how to swim is much more likely to drown than one who does not!

Overuse and injury remain two significant risk factors for *osteoarthritis*. This is a term given to joint disease resulting from wear and tear. Some individuals are more susceptible to it than others, and there may be a hereditary component. Joint disease resulting from injury is strictly localized to the area originally affected. This pattern is called *secondary osteoarthritis*. Commonly affected areas include the knees, hips, and lower back.

Another form of this disorder is idiopathic, possibly with a genetic component, where non-weight-bearing joints are also involved. Thus, we see advanced disease in sites such as the fingers and the base of the thumb along with the knees and hips. This is often seen in elderly women. They present with firm swellings at the distal two joints of the fingers. Some have deviation of the tips of the fingers toward the small fingers in both hands. In both cases, there is wearing down of the joint cartilage over time.

Often, patients experience discomfort in the affected joint during periods of prolonged immobility, such as following sleep or long car trips. The joint feels better once the individual is up and moving. This has been called the *theatre sign*.

The wear and tear is accelerated in many sports as well as certain occupations. For example, racquet sports, football, and basketball, which involve rapid stops, changes in direction, and acceleration, may often result in disabling arthritis in the lower extremities in later life. Unfortunately, certain occupations may also predispose one to this disorder. Carpenters repeatedly lift heavy objects and work with their knees bent for long periods, stressing the joints in the lower extremities. There is also overuse of the small joints of the hands. Similar problems can also appear in the soft tissues that support joints, resulting in inflammation; these are referred to as *tendonitis* or *bursitis*. Others develop chronic low back pain.

A series of adaptive behaviors is seen in individuals with chronic problems of this type. Aggravating activities such as certain sports and hobbies are avoided. An individual with chronic pain in the right knee will carry a heavy briefcase or suitcase in the left hand in order to shift the center of gravity to that side. A cane or walking stick should also be held in the same manner. When there is pain in the dominant shoulder, he or she will learn to perform heavy tasks with the non-dominant hand. Physicians frequently encounter patients who exhibit maladaptive behavior patterns. These patients are highly sensitized to the pain, misuse insurance policies, and develop personality difficulties and over-dependence on painkillers.

The knee joint is particularly vulnerable in all the activities described above. However, obesity still remains the most important risk factor for arthritis in this joint. The knee has two cartilaginous cushions that are prone to damage or tears through overuse or injury. In time, the smooth cartilage covering the ends of the long bones also starts to thin. Following this, abnormal densities appear in the bones underlying the cartilage as well as bony spurs around the joint. The whole joint may appear deformed and enlarged. Ultimately, the ends of the thigh and shinbones almost rest on each other.

Often patients have mild discomfort and stiffness without any swelling at first. The stiffness is worse following periods of rest and improves with activity. Eventually, this progresses to further pain and noticeable swelling. The physician may elect to treat this stage with *anti-inflammatory medications*. Another approach is to aspirate the joint and inject corticosteroids. Joint replacement is an option for many seniors, but knee replacement is still a serious operation involving general anesthesia and several months of recovery.

OUTDOOR PHYSICAL ACTIVITY

Let us look at some other issues regarding outdoor activities in general. We live in highly urbanized environments, with the populations of rural communities shrinking as people migrate into cities. We are facing global warming, expanding holes in the ozone layer, increasing ultraviolet radiation and ozone at ground level, and atmospheric pollution. Hot summer weather increases the generation of harmful smog particles. Smog warnings are now more common than ever in North American cities. These coincide with increased visits to hospital emergency rooms and premature deaths. People suffering from chronic lung or heart problems are affected particularly. The elderly, children, and pregnant women are at increased risk also. During such periods, those who are active outdoors are placing their health at risk. An individual who jogs several kilometers in a smoggy city is sharing air space with hundreds of automobiles. A highly polluted atmosphere also impairs the production of vitamin D in the skin.

Fortunately, the debate on air quality is becoming more and more serious, and major effort is being exerted at the political level as well as by industry. Welcome news in recent years has been the development of more efficient gasoline engines, hybrid vehicles, legislation against large factories using fossil fuels, conservation of forests (which act as sinks for carbon dioxide, a gas that is a significant component of the greenhouse phenomenon), and the use of nuclear energy in homes and industry.

An additional public health concern is prolonged exposure to ultraviolet radiation from the summer sun. There is a clear association of several types of skin cancer with increased exposure, tanning and sunburns. The risk increases in fairer skin types. *Malignant melanoma* is a particularly lethal type of skin cancer that can result from these activities. Prolonged exposure to the sun results in premature aging of the skin, which assumes a thick leathery appearance with wrinkles. It also promotes clouding of the lens of the eye, a condition called *cataracts*. For most people, the majority of their lifetime exposure to outdoor sunlight occurs by age sixteen. After this, the frequency of exposure depends on lifestyle, occupation, and hobbies. Sunblocks are strongly recommended for those who spend significant amounts of time outdoors.

The lawns and fields children play in should be protected from invisible problems such as herbicides and pesticides. Researchers are starting to discover health problems associated with long-term exposure to these agents.

LONGEVITY

If longevity is the main objective of exercise, it is also important to consider the time that must be spent in order to attain this goal. Studies show that a healthy, active lifestyle confers two to three years of additional survival. It is not uncommon to come across individuals who exercise four or five hours weekly on a regular basis. If one were to do this for forty years, say from age fifteen to fifty-five, then one out of those two or three years gained is spent exercising! Clearly, some of us have other priorities.

There are some flaws in this analysis even from a medical point of view that can be illustrated when we examine the other extreme. An individual with a very sedentary lifestyle will have a shorter life span on average. Additionally, this person is more likely to suffer from other medical conditions associated with this lifestyle choice. These disorders may include premature atherosclerosis and diabetes, resulting in high blood pressure, angina, heart attacks, strokes, and kidney disease. These disorders tend to be clinically symptomatic for decades, resulting in suffering and disability before the patient finally succumbs to them.

These issues are important points of discussion with health-care providers. Once goals have been established, the medical approach can be individualized. As discussed before, issues of safety can also be raised. This is important for all age groups. Physicians see too many eye injuries, fractures, and concussions resulting from sports when many of these could be avoided through education and awareness. Competitive sports are a particular concern since there is much less control exerted by any given participant.

Physicians cannot adopt a one-size-fits-all type of approach with their patients. We know that life expectancy is influenced by genetic and environmental factors. Other important contributors, which are not directly related to physical fitness, include sleeping habits, stress levels, family and social support systems, mood disorders, and satisfaction with life in general. Overweight individuals lose an average of three years of life expectancy whereas the obese lose six or seven years.

Premature heart disease was the initial impetus for intensive research, which led to many of our modern medical recommendations. This term specifically refers to the development of cardiovascular problems, that is symptoms of ischemic heart disease and stroke, including death, prior to the age of sixty years. Symptomatic heart disease, including heart attacks, has a profound impact on survival, quality of life, and mental health in these patients who are relatively young. In addition, there is an immeasurable impact on patients' families along with a significant quantitative cost to society in terms of lost productivity. We can conclude that medical research has addressed these problems successfully. Physicians are able to make meaningful health recommendations and use medications appropriately. Interventional cardiologists and cardiovascular surgeons are able to perform rescue procedures with excellent outcomes.

Contrasting with the successful record for heart disease, medical gains in the fight against cancer have been limited. There have been small declines in cancer death rates, in the last five years only, for malignancies in the large bowel, breast, lung and prostate. Death rates from most cancers had been increasing for seventy years prior to this time (the main exceptions were cancers of the stomach and uterus). Since heart disease had been responsible for most deaths by far, it is likely that increasing life expectancy also provides an opportunity for malignancies to develop to symptomatic stages. This is the next great frontier in medical health in affluent countries. Meanwhile, family physicians will continue to try to use evidence-based screening methods to identify cancers in the hope that early detection equals cure.

Personal priorities

The issue of priorities in life is one that many physicians are not comfortable addressing. Part of the reason for this is that they are not trained to deal with this important aspect of life. These issues remain highly personal decisions. The pursuit for physical fitness may have assumed a much lower standing for many individuals. We meet people who are motivated primarily by their careers and status as well as the accumulation of wealth. Others may be caregivers for sick or aged loved ones. Many others are already struggling with poverty, drug addiction, alcoholism, or with other significant medical disorders. Weight control and physical fitness are often lesser priorities with these individuals. They rarely discuss the issue of fitness and fail to follow up if the physician raises the topic. Often, they present after adverse medical consequences of their lifestyle choices have occurred.

A pervasive problem with strategies designed to prolong life expectancy is that they do not address the issue of medical disorders independent of lifestyle. For instance, we can quote statistics that show that a certain change in diet or lifestyle is associated with longevity via reduction in heart disease, stroke, and cancer, yet we cannot begin to address the risks of developing serious neurological disorders such as dementia, multiple sclerosis or Parkinson's disease in that same manner. We do not want to replace a relatively quick manner of dying with a slower more painful or degrading one. Physicians have noted fundamental differences in the reaction that patients have to their medical diagnoses. Patients experience profound disappointment, betrayal and fear with medical problems such as Crohn's disease, neurological diseases and cancer. In contrast, the patient's identity, body image and sense of self-worth are not disturbed to the same degree with heart disease. This phenomenon remains poorly understood by medical doctors.

Physicians do not pretend to have all the answers. Many of us recognize that enormous effort, technology, and revenue are utilized in the latter part of life. More than ninety percent of the revenue spent on medical care is done in the last six months of each individual's life. We also appreciate that we do not want to prolong the dying process using medical technology in all individuals, adding to suffering and hopelessness. Ideally, not only would we like to add years to lives, but also life to years.

When dealing with patients, we find that the pursuit of health and longevity has different meaning at different stages in life. Children can be devastated when they begin to comprehend mortality, and for many this influences the approach to personal health for several decades. Thus, young adults take a keen interest in issues pertaining to physical health. In some cases, this concern continues into middle age, which is also a time for reflection and reconciliation. Eventually, this leads to understanding and acceptance of one's achievements and failures, and the individual is emotionally prepared for the next stage. Finally, most seniors have come to terms with their mortality and a blind pursuit for longevity is no longer their paramount concern. They want physicians to help maintain quality of life, control discomfort, and assist them when age, infirmity, and disease overcome them.

10

Glossary of Medical Terms

Abdomen: the portion of the body extending from the bottom of the rib cage to the hip bones. It contains the stomach, pancreas, liver, spleen, and intestines.

Adenoids: tissue found in the back of the mouth and below the passages of the nose.

Adipose tissue: a collection of cells containing and storing fatty substances. This tissue is found around our internal organs and under the skin.

Adrenaline: also called epinephrine. This hormone is produced in the adrenal gland to stimulate many body functions.

Amino acids: the building blocks of proteins.

Anemia: a lower blood count than normal.

Aneurysm: an abnormal enlargement of a blood vessel that can rupture.

Angina: pain arising from lack of oxygen to the heart.

Angioplasty: opening blockages in arteries using a balloon passed along blood vessels.

Apnea: temporary cessation of breathing.

Appendicitis: acute inflammation of the appendix, which is located at the beginning of the large bowel. This structure is removed surgically when it becomes inflamed or infected.

Arthritis: inflammation of the joint.

Ascitis: presence of fluid in the abdomen, usually related to liver disease.

Atherosclerosis: deposition of yellowish plaques containing cholesterol and other fatty substances on the inner lining of arteries. This interferes with the flow of blood to the organs.

Artery/arteries: thick-walled blood vessels that carry blood away from the heart to other organs of the body. They have the important role of bringing blood rich in oxygen to the tissues.

Autonomic nervous system: part of the nervous system that regulates heart function, breathing, digestion, secretion from glands, and blood flow. We are not normally aware of these functions.

Basal metabolic rate: the minimal energy required to maintain the vegetative functions of the body, such as breathing, circulation of the blood, and body temperature.

Beta-blockers: medications designed to block the stimulation of the heart by adrenaline.

Cancer: abnormal tissue resulting from derangement in shape, function, and growth of cells. It has a tendency to invade nearby structures or travel by the blood supply to invade other tissues.

Calorie: energy content of food. The Calorie written with a large C is equal to 1000 calories or 1 kilocalorie.

Cardiomyopathy: structural abnormality of heart muscle resulting in deranged heart function.

Cataract: clouding of the lens of the eye.

Cholesterol: a fatty substance produced in the body and also found in foods of animal origin. It is an important chemical constituent of blockages found in arteries.

Chronic obstructive pulmonary disease: or COPD. A serious lung disease resulting in loss of lung tissue and irreversible narrowing of the airways. It is further divided into chronic bronchitis and emphysema.

Cirrhosis: end-stage liver disease where normal cells are replaced by scar or fibrous tissue.

Congestive heart failure: inability of the heart to provide adequate flow of nutrients and oxygen to the tissues.

Coronary: pertaining to the heart

Corticosteroid: a synthetic substance resembling or natural substance produced by the adrenal gland. It should not be confused with steroids produced by the reproductive organs.

Crohn's disease: a chronic disease affecting the entire digestive tract resulting in bloody diarrhea, intestinal blockages, and infections.

Cruciate ligament: one of two ligaments found within the knee joint. Together they help to stabilize the knee joint.

Dehydration: the condition resulting from excessive loss of water or fluid from the body.

Dementia: chronic decline in mental function with impairment in memory, insight, and judgment. It is a progressive disease resulting ultimately in an inability of the individual to care for his or her basic needs. There are many causes of dementia.

Depression: a disorder of mood whereby a person reports chronic sadness, hopelessness, fatigue, poor concentration, and an inability to enjoy activities.

Desaturation: decline in the amount of hemoglobin carrying oxygen in the blood.

Diabetes: abnormality in the ability of the body to regulate blood sugar, leading to deficiencies in the tissues. Blood-sugar (glucose) levels are increased but the tissues cannot utilize this substance for energy.

Diverticulosis: pouches formed along the wall of the large bowel that can become inflamed resulting in bleeding and obstruction.

Dyslipidemia: abnormal fat or lipid profile in the blood.

Dysthymia: chronic unhappiness.

Edema: presence of excessive fluid in parts of the body.

Electrocardiogram: ECG or EKG. A record of the electrical activity of the heart produced on the body's surface.

Endothelium: inner lining of blood vessels. It is now recognized as having an important metabolic role.

Epinephrine: another name for adrenaline. This hormone, produced by the adrenal gland, has many stimulatory effects on the body.

Estrogen: the major hormone involved in female maturation and reproduction.

Fatty acids: a type of fat molecule.

Folic acid/folate: a B vitamin involved in the production of blood cells and proper functioning of nerves. It is found in green leafy vegetables.

Gastritis: inflammation of the inner lining of the stomach.

Glucose: the most important form of sugar in the blood.

Hallucination: a sensory perception in the absence of external stimulation. For example, a person may hear a voice when there is no one speaking.

Hemorrhage: bleeding resulting from the rupture of a blood vessel.

Hepatitis: inflammation of the liver due to various insults.

Hirsute: being hairy.

Hormone: a protein or steroid substance produced by one type of cells, carried by the blood stream and having an action on another type of cell.

Hyperglycemia: high blood sugar.

Hypoglycemia: low blood sugar.

Hypertension: high blood pressure. Blood pressure is the force of the blood against the walls of the arteries. It is expressed as two numbers. The upper number reflects the pressure when the heart pumps blood into the arteries and the lower number is the pressure when the heart relaxes.

Idiopathic: of unknown causes.

Insulin: the key hormone regulating blood sugar and fat deposition.

Ischemia/ischemic: lack of oxygen.

Ketones: acidic chemicals produced from fat in uncontrolled diabetes or starvation.

Lactose: sugar found naturally in milk products.

Lactose intolerance: an inability to digest milk sugar resulting in bloating, cramps and diarrhea.

Lateral: away from the midline.

Laxative: a chemical that induces rapid passage of stool through the intestine or bowel.

Legumes: peas, beans, and lentils.

Lipids: another term for fats.

Macrovascular: reference to the larger blood vessels, which conduct blood to organs.

Malignant melanoma: an aggressive type of skin cancer generally presenting as a growing dark spot on the skin.

Medial: towards the midline.

Meniscus: crescent-shaped cartilage cushion in the knee joint.

Menstruation: the female reproductive cycle; more specifically refers to the cyclic flow of blood from the reproductive tract.

Metabolism: a general term given to all the chemical reactions that take place in the body.

Microvascular: reference to the smaller blood vessels of the body that are involved in the exchange of nutrients, oxygen, and carbon dioxide in the tissues.

Morbidity: illness and suffering.

Mortality: death.

Multiple sclerosis: a progressive disease of the nervous system resulting in variable sensory and muscular symptoms. There is a loss of protective insulating sheaths around nerve cells at the microscopic level.

Myocardial infarction: heart attack. The destruction of heart muscle by lack of oxygen.

Osteoarthritis: a disease resulting from a wearing down of or injury to a joint. Some forms appear to have a genetic basis.

Osteoporosis: reduction in the amount of bone in the skeleton leading to easier fractures. It can occur secondary to the loss of estrogen in post-menopausal women. Senile osteoporosis is found in very aged men and women. Osteoporosis is the commonest bone disease in the world.

Ovary: the structure producing the egg as well as female reproductive hormones.

Oxalic acid/oxalate: a substance found in many fruits and vegetables. It is related to vitamin C.

Pancreas: organ involved in production of digestive enzymes and insulin.

Pancreatitis: inflammation of the pancreas due to various factors, such as alcohol, gallstones.

Parathyroid hormone: hormone produced by the parathyroid gland regulating blood and bone calcium. The parathyroid gland is embedded in the thyroid gland.

Parkinson's disease: a progressive disease of the central nervous system resulting in a shuffling gait, rigid facial expression, shaking of the extremities at rest, and finally dementia.

Pernicious anemia: low blood level due to a deficiency of vitamin B12.

Pickwickian syndrome: the association of obesity with breathing impairment, daytime sleepiness, high blood count, failure of the right side of the heart, and increased appetite. The disorder gets its name from a novel by Charles Dickens.

Platelets: small cell-like structures found in blood that are involved in clotting.

Pneumonia: infection in the lungs commonly seen using x-rays.

Potassium: the main component of salt found within cells.

Pubic: genital area.

Pulmonary: pertaining to the lungs.

Quadriceps: the large muscle at the front of the thigh that straightens the knee.

Radial artery: the main artery supplying blood to the hand. Its pulse can be felt at the front of the wrist on the thumb side.

Sign: an abnormality that is observed by the examiner; for example, the physician notices an irregular heart beat when listening to the chest.

Sodium: the main component of salt found in blood. It is also found in table salt.

Stenosis: narrowing.

Stroke: destruction of brain tissue due to lack of oxygen following a blockage or rupture of a blood vessel.

Symptom: an abnormality that the patient reports; for example, "I get short of breath when I lie down."

Syndrome: a cluster of symptoms and signs, sometimes having a common cause.

Tendonitis: inflammation of a tendon. A tendon is a fibrous cord that connects muscle to bone.

Teratogen: an agent that causes physical defects in the developing fetus.

Theatre sign: also called inactivity stiffness or morning stiffness. Joint discomfort following a period of rest. It is a marker of inflammation of the joint.

Thiamine: vitamin B1. A vitamin involved in the production of energy from carbohydrates.

Thrombus: clot formed within blood vessels or the heart. This is the main mechanism whereby blood supply is cut off to a part of an organ.

Thyroid gland: gland located just below the voice box in front of the windpipe. It is involved in regulating body temperature and the rate of metabolism.

Thyroid stimulating hormone: hormone produced at the base of the brain to control the thyroid gland.

Thyroxine: the main hormone produced by the thyroid gland.

Tissue: collection of similar cells performing a specific specialized function.

Tonsils: tissue found at the back part of the mouth. It is part of the lymphatic system.

Triglycerides: a common type of fat found in fat tissue and blood.

Viscera: collective term applied to the internal organs of the body.

Vitamin B12: important for the production of blood cells and proper functioning of the brain and nerves. It acts with folic acid. Vitamin B12 is found in milk and eggs.

Vitamin C: also known as ascorbic acid. A substance found in many fruits and vegetables, especially citrus fruit and tomatoes. Deficiency leads to delayed healing of wounds.

Vitamin D: the major vitamin involved in the regulation of calcium, including uptake from the digestive system and deposition in bone.

Vitamins: a number of unrelated substances found in food essential for proper functioning of chemical processes within cells.

11

List of References

Abelsohn A, D Stieb, MD Sanborn, E Weir, "Identifying and Managing Adverse Environmental Health Effects: 2. Outdoor Air Pollution," *CMAJ.* 166, no. 9 (2002): 1161-1167.

Baker MM, "Anterior Cruciate Ligament Injuries in the Female Athlete," *J Women's Health* 7, no. 3 (1998): 343-349.

Braunwald E, AS Fauci, DL Kasper, SL Hauser, DL Longo, JL Jameson, eds., *Harrison's Principles of Internal Medicine.* 15th ed. New York: The McGraw-Hill Co., Inc, 2001.

Castillo-Duran C, F Cassorla, "Trace Minerals in Human Growth and Development," *J Pediatr Endocrinol Metab.* 12, no. 2, supp. 2 (1999): 589-601.

Chan JM, EL Giovannucci, "Dairy Products, Calcium, and Vitamin D and Risk of Prostate Cancer," *Epidemiol Rev.* 23, no. 1 (2001): 87-92.

Christmas C, RA Anderson, "Exercise and Older Patients: Guidelines for the Clinician," *J Am Geriatr Soc.* 48, no. 3 (2000): 318-324.

Craig WJ, "Iron Status of Vegetarians," *Am J Clin Nutr.* 59 (1994): 1233-1237.

Donovon UM, RS Gibson, "Dietary Intakes of Adolescent Females Consuming Vegetarian, Semi-vegetarian, and Omnivorous Diets," *J Adolesc Health* 18, no. 4 (1996): 292-300.

Drewnowski A, "Fat and Sugar: An Economic Analysis," *J. Nutr.* 133, no. 3 (2003): 838-840.

Drewnowski A, WJ Evans, "Nutrition, physical activity, and quality of life in older adults: summary," *J Gerontol A Biol Sci Med Sci.* 56, no. 2 (2001): 89-94.

Ellsworth JL, LH Kushi, AR Folsom, "Frequent Nut Intake and Risk of Death from Coronary Heart Disease and All Causes in Postmenopausal Women: the Iowa Women's Health Study," *Nutr Metab Cardiovasc Dis.* 11, no. 6 (2001): 372-377.

Feskanich D, WC Willett, GA Colditz, "Calcium, Vitamin D, Milk Consumption, and Hip Fractures: a Prospective Study Among Postmenopausal Women," *Am J Clin Nutr.* 77, no. 2 (2003): 504-511.

Gallagher KI, JM Jakicic, DP Kiel, ML Page, ES Ferguson, BH Marcus, "Impact of Weight-cycling History on Bone Density in Obese Women," *Obes Res.* 10, no. 9 (2002): 896-902.

Gibson RS, JE McKenzie, EL Ferguson, WR Parnell, NC Wilson, DG Russell, "The Risk of Inadequate Zinc Intake in United States and New Zealand Adults," *Nutr Today.* 38, no. 2 (2003): 63-70.

Glimet T, JP Masse, D Kuntz, "Obesity and Arthritis of the Knee," *Rev Rhum Mal Osteoartic.* 57, no. 3 (1990): 207-209.

Gutierrez M, M Akhavan, L Jovanovic, CM Peterson, "Utility of a Short-term 25% Carbohydrate Diet on Improving Glycemic Control in Type 2 Diabetes Mellitus," *J Am Coll Nutr.* 17, no. 6 (1998): 595-600.

Health Canada. *Nutrition for a Healthy Pregnancy: National Guidelines for the Childbearing Years. Ottawa: Minister of Public Works and Government Services Canada.* 1999.

Hu FB, WC Willett, "Optimal Diets for Prevention of Coronary Heart Disease," *JAMA.* 288, no. 20 (2002): 2569-2578.

Kalkwarf HJ, JC Khoury, BP Lanphear, "Milk Intake During Childhood and Adolescence, Adult Bone Density, and Osteoporotic Fractures in US Women," *Am J Clin Nutr.* 77, no.1 (2003): 257-265.

Katschinski B, RF Logan, M Edmond, MJ Langman, "Smoking and Sugar Intake are Separate but Interactive Risk Factors for Crohn's Disease," *Gut.* 29, no.9 (1988): 1202-1206.

Kimm SY, NW Glynn, AM Kriska, BA Barton, SS Kronsberg, SR Daniels, PB Crawford, ZI Sabry, K Liu, "Decline in Physical Activity in Black Girls and

White Girls During Adolescence," *N Engl J Med.* 347, no. 10 (2002): 709-715.

Knekt P, R Jarvinen, R Seppanen, E Pukkala, A Aromaa, "Intake of Dairy Products and the Risk of Breast Cancer," *Br J Cancer.* 73, no. 5 (1996): 687-691.

Lakka HM, DE Laaksonen, TA Lakka, LK Niskanen, E Kumpusalo, J Tuomilehto, JT Salonen, "The Metabolic Syndrome and Total and Cardiovascular Disease Mortality in Middle-aged Men," *JAMA.* 288, no. 21 (2002): 2709-2716.

Lau EM, T Kwok, J Woo, SC Ho, "Bone Mineral Density in Chinese Elderly Female Vegetarians, Vegans, Lacto-vegetarians and Omnivores," *Eur J Clin Nutr.* 52, no. 1 (1998): 60-64.

Lichtenstein AH, LM Ausman, SM Jalbert, EJ Schaefer, "Effects of Different Forms of Dietary Hydrogenated Fats on Serum Lipoprotein Cholesterol Levels," *N Engl J Med.* 340, no. 25 (1999): 1933-1940.

Lipton AJ, D Gozal, "Treatment of Obstructive Sleep Apnea in Children: Do We Really Know How?" *Sleep Med Rev.* 7, no. 1 (2003): 61-80.

Mahan LK, S Escott-Stump ed. *Krause's Food, Nutrition, and Diet Therapy.* 10th ed. Philadelphia: W.B. Saunders Co., 2000.

Mahan LK, MT Arlin ed. *Krause's Food, Nutrition, and Diet Therapy.* 8th ed. Philadelphia: W.B. Saunders Co., 1992.

Manson JE, P Greenland, AZ LaCroix, ML Stefanick, CP Mouton, A Oberman, MD Perri, DS Sheps, MB Pettinger, DS Siscovick, "Walking Compared to Vigorous Exercise for the Prevention of Cardiovascular Events in Women," *N Engl J Med.* 347, no. 10 (2002): 716-725.

Marshall KG. *Mosby's Family Practice Sourcebook. Evidence-based Emphasis.* St. Louis: Mosby, Inc. 1999.

McElduff P, AJ Dobson, "How Much Alcohol and How Often? Population Based Case-control Study of Alcohol Consumption and Risk of a Major Coronary Event," *BMJ.* 314, no. 7088 (1997): 1159-1164.

Meckling KA, M Gauthier, R Grubb, J Sanford, "Effects of a Hypocaloric, Low-carbohydrate Diet on Weight Loss, Blood Lipids, Blood Pressure, Glucose Tolerance, and Body Composition in Free-living Overweight Women," *Can J Physiol Pharmacol.* 80, no. 11 (2002): 1095-1105.

Menotti A, D Kromhout, H Blackburn, R Fidanza, R Buzina, A Nissinen, "Food Intake Patterns and 25-Year Mortality from Coronary Heart Disease: Cross-cultural Correlations in the Seven Countries Study. The Seven Countries Study Research Group," *Eur J Epidemiol.* 15, no. 6 (1999): 507-515.

Mittleman MA, M Maclure, GH Toffler, JB Sherwood, RJ Goldberg, JE Muller, "Triggering of Acute Myocardial Infarction by Heavy Physical Exertion. Protection Against Triggering by Regular Exertion. Determinants of Myocardial Infarction Onset Study Investigators," *N Eng J Med.* 329, no. 23 (1993): 1677-1683.

Mojzisova G, M Kuchta, "Dietary Flavonoids and Risk of Coronary Heart Disease," *Physiol Res.* 50, no. 6 (2001): 529-535.

Morgan JM, K Horton, D Reese, C Carey, K Walker, DM Capuzzi, "Effects of Walnut Consumption as Part of a Low-fat, Low-cholesterol Diet on Serum Cardiovascular Risk Factors," *Int J Vitam Nutr Res.* 72, no. 5 (2002): 341-347.

Ornish D, LW Scherwitz, JH Billings, SE Brown, KL Gould, TA Merritt, S Sparler, WT Armstrong, TA Ports, RL Kirkeeide, C Hogeboom, RJ Brand, "Intensive Lifestyle Changes for Reversal of Coronary Heart Disease," *JAMA.* 280, no. 23 (1998): 2001-2007.

Peeters A, JJ Barendregt, F Willekens, JP Mackenbach, A Al Mamun, L Bonneux, "Obesity in Adulthood and its Consequences for Life Expectancy: a Life-table Analysis," *Ann Intern Med.* 138, no. 1 (2003): 24-32.

Rehm J, CT Sempos, M Trevisan, "Average Volume of Alcohol Consumption, Patterns of Drinking and Risk of Coronary Heart Disease-a Review," *J Cardiovasc Risk.* 10, no. 1 (2003): 15-20.

Sacks FM, D Ornish, B Rosner, S McLanahan, WP Castelli, EH Kass, "Plasma Lipoprotein Levels in Vegetarians. The Effect of Ingestion of Fats from Dairy Products," *JAMA.* 254, no. 10 (1998): 1337-1441.

Samaha FF, N Iqbal, P Seshadri, KL Chicano, DA Daily, J McGrory, T Williams, M Williams, EJ Gracely, L Stern, "A Low-carbohydrate as Compared with a Low-fat diet in Severe Obesity," *N Engl J Med.* 348, no. 21 (2003): 2074-2081.

Sandberg AS, "Bioavailability of Minerals in Legumes," *Br J Nutr.* 88, suppl 3 (2002): S281-S285.

Schmitz KH, DR Jacobs, CP Hong, J Steinberger, A Moran, AR Sinaiko, "Association of Physical Activity with Insulin Sensitivity in Children," *Int J Obes Relat Metab Disord.* 26, no. 10 (2002): 1310-1316.

Shils ME, JA Olson, M Shike ed. *Modern Nutrition in Health and Disease.* 8th ed. Philadelphia: Lea and Febiger, 1994.

Shin MH, MD Holmes, SE Hankinson, K Wu, GA Colditz, WC Willet, "Intake of Dairy Products, Calcium, and Vitamin D and Risk of Breast Cancer," *J Natl Cancer Inst.* 94, no. 17 (2002): 1301-1310.

Smolander J, V Louhevaara, E Ahonen, J Polari, T Klen, "Energy Expenditure and Clearing Snow: a Comparison of Shovel and Snow Pusher," *Ergonomics.* 38, no. 4 (1995): 749-753.

Sorof J, S Daniels, "Obesity Hypertension in Children: a Problem of Epidemic Proportions," *Hypertension.* 40, no. 4 (2002): 441-441.

Stampfer MJ, FB Hu, JE Manson, EB Rimm, WC Willet, "Primary Prevention of Coronary Heart Disease in Women through Diet and Lifestyle," *N Engl J Med.* 343, no. 1 (2000):16-22.

Tanasescu M, MF Leitzmann, EB Rimm, WC Willet, MJ Stampfer, FB Hu, "Exercise Type and Intensity in Relation to Coronary Heart Disease in Men," *JAMA* 288, no. 16 (2002):1994-2000.

Toth AP, FA Cordasco, "Anterior Cruciate Ligament Injuries in the Female Athlete," *J Gend Specif Med.* 4, no. 4 (2001): 25-34.

Tuomilehto J, J Lindstrom, JG Eriksson, TT Valle, H Hamalainen, P Ilanne-Parikka, S Keinanen-Kiukaanniemi, M Laakso, A Louheranta, M Rastas, V Salminen, M Uusitupa; Finnish Diabetes Prevention Study Group, "Prevention of Type 2 Diabetes Mellitus by Changes in Lifestyle Among Subjects with Impaired Glucose Tolerance," *N Engl J Med.* 344, no. 18 (2001): 1343-1350.

UKPDS Group, "Tight Blood Pressure Control and Risk of Macrovascular and Microvascular Complications in Type 2 Diabetes: UKPDS 38," *BMJ.* 317, no. 7160 (1998): 703-713.

Wasserman D, R Mangels. *Simply Vegan.* 3rd ed. Baltimore: The Vegetarian Resource Group, 1999.

Wing RR, JO Hill, "Successful Weight Loss Maintenance," *Annu Rev Nutr.* 21 (2001): 323-341.

0-595-28103-6

Printed in the United States
125571LV00015B/282/A